D1636690

Looking Back: Memoir of a Psychoanalyst

ALSO BY PAUL ORNSTEIN

Focal Psychotherapy — An Example of Applied Psychoanalysis (with Michael and Enid Balint)

The Search for the Self: Selected Writings of Heinz Kohut

ALSO BY HELEN EPSTEIN

A Jewish Athlete: Swimming Against Stereotype in 20th Century Europe

Archivist on a Bicycle: Jiří Fiedler

Children of the Holocaust

Joe Papp: An American Life

Meyer Schapiro: Portrait of an Art Historian

Music Talks: the lives of classical musicians

Tina Packer Builds A Theater

Where She Came From: A Daughter's Search for Her Mother's History

Looking Back: Memoir of a Psychoanalyst

by Paul H. Ornstein

with Helen Epstein

PLUNKETT LAKE PRESS

Lexington, Massachusetts

ISBN: 978-0-9614696-3-4

Published by Plunkett Lake Press, 2015
www.plunkettlakepress.com

Simultaneously published by Plunkett Lake Press as an electronic book:
www.plunkettlakepress.com/lbmp.html

CONTENTS

PREFACE	7
ONE ~ Birth to 1939	13
TWO ~ Seminary and Psychoanalysis	31
THREE ~ 1944	47
FOUR ~ Germany	69
FIVE ~ United States	83
SIX ~ Cincinnati	93
SEVEN ~ Chicago	113
EIGHT ~ Life outside Analysis	127
NINE ~ Kohut	139
TEN ~ Retirement and Family	155
AFTERWORD by Charles Fenyvesi	169
ACKNOWLEDGMENTS	175
GLOSSARY	177
PUBLICATIONS by Paul Ornstein	180

PREFACE

I have two distinct sets of memories of Hajdúnánás, the exquisitely dusty town near the great plain of Hortobágy in the east of Hungary where I lived until I was fifteen years old. As a psychoanalyst, I am aware that memories are thought to be newly assembled each time one reaches into one's mind to get hold of them. My memories of the town in which I spent my first fifteen years, however, always emerge with identical images and identical emotions, as if I had to fix these memories in my mind, hold on to them, never to lose them.

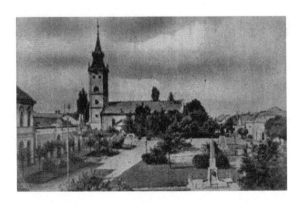

In my mind, the town of about 18,000 northwest of

Debrecen is always the same, every inch familiar: its streets, its two parks, its bookstore, theater and cinema; two Jewish bakeries; three pharmacies; the post office. There is no hospital — you have to go to Debrecen for that — but a kind of clinic where midwives help women give birth.

On Sundays, the Protestants attend the large church and the Catholics a smaller one. On *Shabbat*, the Hasidim walk to a small *shul* and everyone else, including my family, to a large synagogue with a courtyard. There is an old "Jewish Street" near the synagogue but by the time I was born, the Jewish population lived all over town.

There are few cars in the Hajdúnánás of my childhood. People going to and from the train station travel by horse-drawn carriage. We have electricity and a gramophone on which we listen to cantorial music but no hot water, no telephone, no radio. Six days a week, the town center is vibrant with commerce. In the 1920s and 1930s, Jews own many of the shops and there are three Jewish doctors. The people do not yet boycott any of them.

My family is still whole; my small Jewish community is intact. There are about 250 Jewish families.

My closest friend Steve Hornstein and I go to *cheder* together at six in the morning six days a week. On *Shabbat*, it's as if the world stops. On Friday nights, we dress for synagogue and my father and I walk to services together. On the Sabbath day, we stop at my maternal grandparents' house on the way home. I stop going to services on Saturdays after I enter Gymnasium, because my Hungarian school meets six days a week. But out of respect for my observant grandparents, I observe the Sabbath commandment and do not carry anything; a woman employed by my parents carries my books.

The routines of our quiet town allow us the illusion that we are protected against the growing hostility of its people. We are accustomed to garden-variety Hungarian anti-semitism; the Nazis will transform it into an unprecedented, murderous kind.

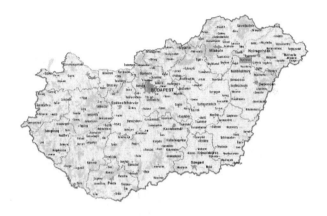

My second set of memories dates from February 1945, after the Russian liberation of Hungary. Even as the war continued west of us, I returned to Hajdúnánás, in search of my family — and found almost no one I knew. My family was gone. Many of the formerly Jewish owned stores were boarded up. To me, Hajdúnánás was now a repulsive ghost-town! Of the 250 Jewish families — about 1,250 souls — no more than fifty would return.

The town center no longer seemed vibrant; our Jewish cemetery was partly destroyed; the marble tombstones were stolen — others overturned, some broken. Our Nazified former neighbors had vandalized everything Jewish, including our graves.

I later found out that as soon as the town's Jews were

marched to the railway station and made to board the cattle cars to Auschwitz, the local population had stolen anything that they were forced to leave behind. The locals began to do this a few weeks earlier, when the Jews had to leave their own homes and move to the ghetto. The Jews had been lulled into thinking that it would be a temporary stay; the Gentiles knew better.

I roamed the town for three days in February of 1945, almost in a daze, trying in vain to find information about my family and my library, unable to suppress recurrent images of what it must have been like for my mother and three brothers to live through their stay in the ghetto and their final journey. Sometimes, I burst out crying as I tried to piece together what happened to my family and the community before their deportation to Auschwitz. No one yet knew the magnitude of the devastation.

I went to the synagogue, hoping for news and found Steve Hornstein among those who returned. I met Steve at the age of four and from that time on we were best friends. Finding each other alive gave both of us some relief from the pain of not finding anyone from our own families. We then found other young Jewish men who had returned. They seemed to feel powerful now, and behaved as though they were in charge of the town. These young Jews took matters into their own hands and told Steve and me that we should go to City Hall, where the basement was being used to jail the local Nazis. They said we would find one of our former teachers there. I was hoping he might know what had happened to my books.

As we walked down to the basement, I saw an old man who had been one of my teachers. He appeared pleased to see us. He must have hoped we would help him get out of there. He had no idea that we had been urged to go there and beat him up. I could not see myself doing that. When he reached out his hand to me for a handshake, I took his hand and shook it. Steve had a hard time forgiving me. I myself wished I had not done it.

Steve was determined to remain in Hungary and go to medical school at the university in the nearby city of Debrecen. I was determined to go to Palestine. Rumor had it that one could get there from Romania, so I set out for Bucharest.

The rumor turned out to be false and I had to remain in Europe for several more years — but I would succeed in turning this painful fact to my advantage, guided, deep down, by my favorite Hebrew mantra: "*Gam zu l'tovah*" ("Even this can turn out for the good"). And it did.

ONE ~ Birth to 1939

I was born on the eve of Passover, on April 4, 1924. The birth of a first child is a significant moment for all parents, but on the eve of Passover, orthodox Jews remember that Jewish first-born sons were spared on that night in Egypt when, according to religious texts, the God of the Israelites inflicted the tenth plague on the Egyptians by smiting their first born sons. As far back as I can remember I had to accompany my father to the synagogue at dawn on the day before Passover, in order to participate in the thanksgiving prayer for the Jewish first-born sons having been spared.

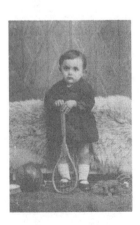

My father, Lajos Ornstein, was an orthodox Jew and a Zionist, more liberal than most of the Jewish community. Even as a child, I knew how much he wanted to take his family to live in Palestine, but didn't have the money to do it, and felt stuck in Hajdúnánás. I knew this from the conversations we used to have every Sabbath, as we walked together back and forth from synagogue. Those walks were wonderful opportunities to learn things.

For example, I remember asking my father about the 2,000-year-old Jewish tradition of breaking the glass at the wedding ceremony. That custom always had a particular fascination for me. I knew it was supposed to remind us of the destruction of the Temple in Jerusalem and all the collective losses in our history. But why should we recall that sadness at the height of joy and happiness? I searched for an ancient *midrash* to find the answer but didn't find one. Then I asked my father, who said, "The Rabbis must have thought that, if we recall the sadness that is connected with the loss of the Temple, we shall feel our joy and happiness at the wedding all the more intensely."

"But then, why choose to remember the loss of the Temple in Jerusalem," I asked him. "Why not remember some of our own losses and sadness?"

"In their wisdom," my father answered patiently, "the Rabbis wanted to connect each and every one of us individually to earlier generations and to our collective historical past." The way I would put it today is that the Rabbis understood that we needed a cohesive group-self to support each individual self. Traditions. Create a collective continuity, whereas each of us has only a very limited lifespan.

I admired my father immensely. He was born in 1896 on Ohatpusztakócs, an estate not far from Hajdúnánás, where his father was the estate manager. That was a job rather frequent for Jews in Hungary of the time. When he was about six years old, the family moved to Nánás so that my father could have a Jewish education. He grew up in a period sometimes seen as the "golden age" of Hungarian Jews, when many Jews assimilated into Hungarian culture. His family spoke Hungarian at home along with some Yiddish and provided him with both a religious and a secular education.

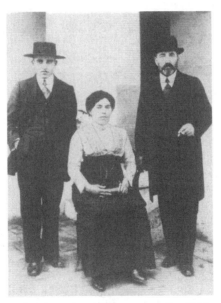

Lajos Ornstein with his parents circa 1914

He attended two famous *yeshivot* for Judaic studies, one

in Hegyalja-Mád, the other in Bratislava. For his secular studies, he attended the "Business Academy" in Miskolc, where he graduated with the equivalent of an MBA. He read voraciously — newspapers, books, magazines — and was revered in the Jewish community for his knowledge of Jewish as well as secular matters.

My father was known as a remarkable orator and was often asked to speak on national holidays in the synagogue, when the speech had to be delivered in Hungarian, and not in Yiddish, in deference to visiting officials of the City Government who might attend.

He had an impressive and unusual linguistic style. His use of apt metaphors, richly interspersed with Biblical and Talmudic quotations as well as with references to classic Hungarian and world literature, made his speeches memorable to me. He could also easily complete any cross-word puzzle. One time, I was maybe ten or eleven, he quoted something to me from the Bible as we were walking, and I asked him: "Will I know as much as you do if I go to rabbinical school?"

He said, "You will know a lot more than I do."

Comments like these left me with good feelings, both about him and about my own future.

Family history had it that, after serving as an officer for the Austro-Hungarian army in World War I, he worked for Grossman-Furth, a distant relative and wholesaler in Czechoslovakia, as a book-keeper. My father was supposed to have ultimately inherited the business. But my grandfather became ill and my father returned to Hungary. I also know that he somehow came to own a bank in his early twenties and lost it in the 1929 stock market crash. He never recovered from that loss emotionally or financially. His later business ventures were not successful, and he became a book-keeper at a flour mill and a tax adviser, using his considerable knowledge in these and other business-related legal issues.

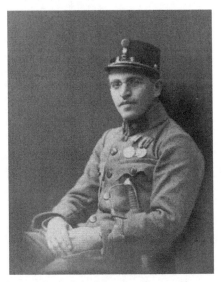

Paul Ornstein's father in officer uniform

My father had such a remarkable memory that he could recall later in life exactly what he had read, where he had read it, or where to look it up. It all seemed to be at his fingertips. I thought I would never be able to reach his level of knowledge. The breadth of it encompassed the Judaic *and* the secular fields, and that was what I, and many other people, most admired.

In 1923, Lajos Ornstein married my mother Frida Cziment, and settled in her hometown of Hajdúnánás, where they would raise five children — myself, my sister Judit, and my brothers Zoltán, Tibor, and László.

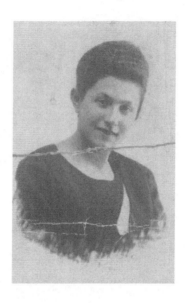

My mother was a beautiful woman; smart, decisive, practical, and devoted to the family. She was the third oldest daughter of a successful wheat merchant in Hajdúnánás. She had two older sisters, two younger brothers and a younger sister. Her formal education ended — as was usual for Jewish girls in the provinces at that time — after completing elementary school but she continued learning at home, with her husband and her children.

She educated herself by reading. I recall her telling me about articles in the high-brow magazines that she devoured, especially one, called *Múlt és Jövő*, "Past and

Future," devoted to Jewish history, literature, archeology, biblical studies and Zionist ideals. I also became a reader of *Múlt és Jövő* in my teens and love to read it to this day, whenever I can get hold of any post World War II issues.

Reading permeated our household and contributed greatly to our pride in who we were. Mother enthusiastically followed my father's activities and interests and could often recite parts of his speeches by heart. She also followed all of her children's schooling and learned along with us as we moved from grade school through the higher levels of learning in the Gymnasium. When I was eight or nine years old, there was an event in the evening when I had to recite a poem. I remember my mother sitting in the front row of the audience and prompting me when I paused and forgot a line. I don't remember ever being punished, hit or spanked. Perhaps we were all very good children or our parents were particularly tolerant parents.

My parents had a traditional Jewish marriage. In those years, a wife and mother was kept busy with everything from tending the fireplace, heating water, preparing food, cleaning, sewing and darning. She had a more "activist" attitude towards the world and the struggle to make a decent living than my father's more passive, "fatalist" one. He was extremely hard-working too and made sure that all of us got into the Gymnasium — hard as it was to finance this from a meager income. But Hajdúnánás was no place for him to make the best use of all his talents — he would have had to look elsewhere.

Mother's energy and good relations with the peasants helped her to procure food when rationing began and the Jewish population began to be isolated. She was "more of *this* world," a doer. He was more "contemplative," a thinker and a bookworm. As I write this, I also realize that he could do and did a lot for others (e.g., staved off bankruptcies or helped others rebound from such calamities) but not for himself.

The tension between my mother's activism and my father's fatalism was palpable in our household. She admired his mind but could not understand why someone that bright couldn't make more money. She was a little nudgy; she felt he should be more entrepreneurial. Her side of the family was doing pretty well financially, while my father was not cut out to be a businessman. That tension between them was chronic: the only time you didn't feel it was from Friday to Saturday night, on *Shabbat.*

That tension, however, only rarely affected the child-centered atmosphere of our home. Both my parents were very loving towards their children. It is this aspect of my family and my "privilege" as the first-born, I believe, that contributed to the sturdiness of my self-esteem. Future adversity could not shake this foundation.

My earliest memories go back to my sister Judit's birth, when I was nearly two and a half years old. I was with a playmate in the living room while the midwife delivered her in the bedroom. I heard strange, anguished noises, periodic screaming and recall seeing a pail of bloody water (with the placenta) brought out of the bedroom by the midwife's helper. I don't recall having been frightened by any of this because my father announced with a beaming expression that I now had a little sister. When I was old enough to ask where babies came from, the stork-story did not impress me because I remembered the mysterious goings-on in and around the bedroom. The birth of my three other siblings, Zoli (two years later), Tibi (four years later) and Laci (ten years later) no longer took place at home, all of them were delivered at the "Stefania" — the small local clinic.

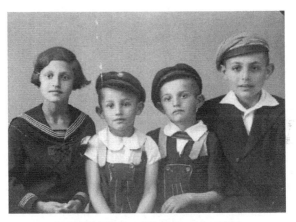

Judit, Tibi, Zoli and Paul Ornstein, 1935

Starting at the age of three and continuing to age five I attended a non-denominational kindergarten. Later, parallel with the four years of grade school, I went to *cheder*, or Hebrew school. My day began at six. I was in cheder from 6:30 to 8:00, then in secular school, then home for lunch for two hours. Then I went back to Hebrew School form 4:00 to 6:00. I did well enough to be able to enter the co-educational Hajdúnánás Gymnasium after the fourth grade, at the age of 10, and spend the next five years there.

Most of the Jewish boys in town attended *yeshiva* but my family wanted me to have both a secular and a Jewish education like my father had had. In 1935, I entered the new and different world of the Gymnasium, not all of it pleasant. Most of my thirty-one classmates were Protestants; a few of them were Catholics; one was Jewish.

I stopped wearing *tzitzit* around this time because we changed clothing for gymnastics, it would have been noticed, and I didn't want any more troubles than I already had.

At the beginning of Gymnasium, in 1935-36, I had several non-Jewish friends. We walked home together but we never went into each other's homes.

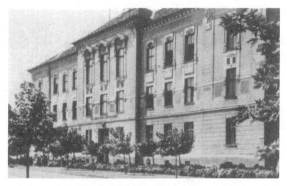

The Hajdúnánás Gymnasium

By the late 1930s, overt anti-semitism became more of the norm and I had a steadily dwindling number of non-Jewish friends. Many took the Nazi-German side and rooted for Hitler, often taunting me that the coming war would be the end of the Jews. What hurt me more than the taunting was something else: in our co-educational class there were ten girls, one more beautiful than the other. During school hours there was no chance to socialize; outside of school even less so. Therefore I could only *imagine* a romantic involvement with two of them (at different times) at a distance. Once I overheard two of the girls whispering to each other that they could like me, but that was impossible because I was Jewish. That did not stop my "being in love" in fantasy.

During those years, fantasizing was a part of my life in another realm too. As anti-semitism became more vocal in our community, I dreamed about escaping from it all by moving to Palestine. I pictured myself being able to outfox the hostile student groups, if directly attacked — unrealistic as that was under the circumstances. It was never one against one, but many against one.

I have a vivid memory of one of the yearly one-day outings by train to a nearby playing field. The entire student body (more than three-hundred of us) and most of the Gymnasium teachers participated. I was 13, a member of the third year class. There were many sports activities at the outing, a picnic lunch and a guided tour of the nearby forest by the Zoology and Botany teacher to identify various forms of vegetation.

Everyone was asked to bring his own lunch-box. In the middle of the lunch, six of my classmates got hold of me, pinned me down to the ground and tried to push a piece of bacon fat into my mouth, to make me eat the most forbidden, non-kosher food. I resisted with all my strength and they could not open my mouth; they only succeeded in touching my teeth with the bacon. One teacher witnessed this from afar but did not intervene.

I knew then that this was a bad omen. Although my classmates behaved as though this were a prank, I realized that there would be no official intervention when similar "teasing" degenerated into bloody attacks. I often reflected on what was behind their trying to force me to eat bacon. I now believe that they resented my insistence on being different; my adhering to and guarding our dietary laws and therefore not participating with them in "breaking bread." After I learned some psychology, I understood that my not eating what they ate was an affront to their self-regard. For me, keeping my mouth closed was an assertion of mine, even at a time when I no longer adhered so strictly to the dietary laws. I refused to concede an inch to their demand and force.

One other example is still vivid in my memory. The people we rented a house from at one time were reasonably well-to-do peasants. They were a likeable family, right next door, with two daughters, slightly older than me. My mother liked to spend time with Mrs. P. exchanging recipes and gossip, and I liked to visit their daughters. Each year, in the fall — as was customary in such peasant families — they slaughtered a pig and had a large feast for their neighbors who helped them in the slaughter and the preparation of the food. We were always invited but, of course, we could not eat anything. All of their food was forbidden to us. Yet, year after year, they kept asking us whether there was anything on the richly-set tables that we were permitted to eat. Despite knowing that it was religiously forbidden to us, they experienced our abstinence as a personal rejection.

I noticed these things, reflected on them, but did not find an explanation then. I was always interested in how other people's minds worked and also in understanding certain things in myself. That may explain my gravitating toward psychoanalysis before I even knew what it was.

I experienced in my teenage years a certain degree of shyness, a lack of ability to approach girls unselfconsciously and with ease. I could not then account for this, but I was curious about its origin and meaning. I eventually overcame my shyness to a degree, but without resolving its inner dynamics, by turning to a study of graphology.

To better understand the girls and what they wanted, I asked for samples of their handwriting and, using the two or three graphology books I had acquired, tried to analyze it. I also tried to analyze my own. Graphology was my first systematic effort, I think, to try to understand my own inner life and that of other people. I bought two or three books by Klara Goldzieher, the most famous Hungarian graphologist of the time. My father laughed at graphology, but I trusted it. I thought handwriting could really tell you something about a person.

I don't know what drew Jews to graphology but some of the most prominent graphologists in Europe at the time were Jews. Hypnosis was another subject that interested me and was also very popular at the time.

Books offered me another way of getting to know the deeper layers of other people's personalities (along with my own) and it gave me something serious to talk about with the girls. I also enjoyed reading poetry, novels and biographies. To a great extent, my close friendship (and competition) with Steve Hornstein, who was more direct and uninhibited with girls, also helped me overcome my shyness. I didn't want to be left behind. A couple of times, we even were attracted to the same girls.

Before the age of 12, Steve and I also had a business partnership. Both my grandfathers received business mail as did our fathers, so we found a stamp collector and sold him stamps that we steamed and dried. We used the money to buy ice cream, *kremes* (Napoleons) from the bakery, and movie tickets on Saturday nights. That is where I saw my first German and American movies.

I finished the fifth year at the Gymnasium in June 1939. The first anti-Jewish laws had been passed in the Hungarian Parliament a year earlier, making it a crime for Gentiles to employ Jews. By 1939, my father could not officially continue his tax-consulting and book-keeping for the non-Jewish flour mills in Hajdúnánás. One was owned by a corporation; the other by an individual, who continued to employ my father in secret, part-time. He took a new job at the Jewish Community but the pay was much lower and he could no longer afford my tuition at the Gymnasium and the education of my siblings.

My friend Steve Hornstein remained in his class as the only Jew. The fact that we chose to attend the Gymnasium rather than *yeshiva* had, all along, been regarded with disapproval by the Jewish community and that had brought us close together. But by the summer of 1939, our interests diverged. Steve was determined to stay on and graduate from the Hajdúnánás Gymnasium. I was determined to go to Palestine that fall or else continue my studies at the Franz Josef National Rabbinical Seminary, where tuition and board were free and I could receive both a secular and a Jewish education.

The Orthodox rabbis were very much against this seminary since the language of instruction there was Hungarian, and it was very much outside the control of the orthodox establishment. The Emperor Franz Josef was largely responsible for its establishment in 1877 and had long supported it. The Seminary promoted an alternative to orthodoxy, called Neolog Judaism among its students. When we graduated, we would obtain rabbinical positions but it was understood that we were going into liberal congregations.

That summer of 1939, I prepared myself for either

Palestine or Budapest. I was the only Jewish teenager from Hajdúnánás to take the train to a Zionist youth camp in the beautiful Mátra mountains about three hours away. The camp was run by the non-religious movement *HaShomer HaTzair* on property owned by a Jew. We slept in tents, harvested wheat, prepared for life in Palestine in a program called *hachsharah*. The plan was to travel to London in the fall, and then go on youth *aliyah* from there.

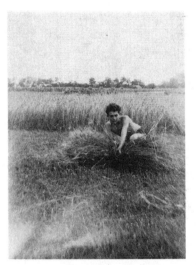

Paul harvesting wheat in 1939

I was very familiar with the history of the Jews in Hungary. I knew that Jews had lived in Hungary prior to the arrival of the Magyars. The Romans found them already there when they conquered the territory. The persecution of the Jews began around the first millennium when King Stephen I converted the Magyars to Christianity while the Jews refused conversion. From then on, the history of the Jews in Hungary was punctuated by pogroms, massacres, and expulsions. They were invited back when needed to lift the economic conditions of the impoverished country. The sequence would be repeated again and again with longer or shorter intervals.

The period 1849 to 1914 is regarded as the Golden Age of Hungarian Jewry. Franz Josef was then Monarch of the Austro-Hungarian Empire, sometimes called the Hapsburg Empire or the "Dual Monarchy of Austria and Hungary." During that time, Jews established financial institutions and large-scale industrial concerns, modernized agriculture, made noteworthy contributions to art, literature, science, medicine, and the law. While assimilation increased, so did the Jews' attention to their own history and culture. Large numbers of Jews fought in the First World War for Austria-Hungary with enthusiasm and bravery, including my father.

This symbiosis, however, was short-lived. The Empire lost the war, was divided, and a bloody Communist regime came to power. Since many of the leaders of this regime were Jews, Admiral Horthy's counter-revolution targeted the Jews as scapegoats. I was born into a country where Jews no longer lived as equals under the law.

By the late 1930s, most Hungarian Jews had given up on an earlier generation's hope of assimilating into Hungarian society. I was fortunate to have grown up with Zionist ideals. For my generation, Zionism provided an emotional antidote to discrimination, episodic harassment, and severe economic hardship. So, for us, it was easy to renounce the Hungarian patriotism of the Hapsburg generations of Jews, to nurture a strong Zionist identification, and to look to the future outside the borders of Hungary.

After that summer of 1939, I never saw anyone from that Zionist camp again. There were rumors of a war starting in Europe and it was impossible for me to get to London. After I returned home, I prepared for my second option, the rabbinical school entrance examination. On August 31, 1939, I took the then 12-hour overnight train from Hajdúnánás to Budapest. When I arrived on September 1, 1939, I learned that Germany had invaded Poland.

TWO ~ Seminary and Psychoanalysis

At the age of fifteen and a half, on the day the Second World War broke out, I was preoccupied by the entrance examination at the Rabbinical Seminary.

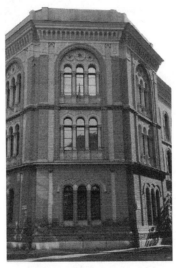

Franz Josef National Rabbinical Seminary

For me, the transition from small, dusty Hajdúnánás to

the great metropolis of Budapest was shocking. I was overwhelmed by the sights and sounds of the city as I walked from the train station to the rabbinical school. I felt well prepared to be examined in Latin, the entire Torah, and 12 or 14 pages of Talmud. A friend, who was already a student there, advised me to put on a *tzitzit*, the ritual garment with fringes that religious Jews wear over their undershirts and under their shirts. I had stopped wearing it by 1939, but now I took the friendly advice, went to the bathroom and slipped the borrowed garment on under my shirt.

I then went into a classroom with two Rabbis. One was old, small, and ugly, and didn't speak Hungarian well; the second was younger with a resounding baritone voice: a Rabbi from a large town. Strangely enough, given the secular orientation of the Seminary, he asked me, "Do you have *tzitzit*?" just as my friend had warned. The older man broke in before I could answer yes and said in a patronizing way, "You don't ask a boy from Hajdúnánás if he wears *tzitzit*!"

Being discovered without *tzitzit* would have been a disaster. The Seminary could have refused me and I would have been forced to learn a trade. Reflecting on this today, I find it interesting that the Seminary, which claimed to be liberal, would have insisted on such an archaic tradition.

My examination went very well; I was admitted. There was no tuition, no charge for the dormitory, and a free breakfast and lunch daily. I could live in Budapest and pursue my education, that otherwise might have had to be interrupted.

I read that the war began on that day in the newspaper headlines. But, at 15, I had no idea of the impact that it would have on my life. First of all, I did not feel that Hungary was my country. I grew up in a Zionist household, wanting to live in Palestine; I didn't feel Hungarian. There seemed to be no immediate threat to us as Jews, although some people with money and foresight began to leave the country. Hungary was Germany's ally: why would Hitler attack us? And sure enough, until 1944, he didn't. During those years while we were studying at the Rabbinical Seminary we were busy with our studies, absorbed in our own lives, and thought the war would blow over.

In those years before 1944, we heard stories of what was happening elsewhere in Europe and thought they were exaggerations. The need to deny was powerful. But there was also the fact that people like my father, who had served in the Austro-Hungarian Army, thought that the Russians might be more dangerous to us than the Germans. He had known the Germans during the First World War and thought Germany was a highly civilized nation.

For me, in September of 1939, the big news was that I was one of twelve boys accepted to the Seminary. The move might have been overwhelming and anxiety-provoking, if not for the protective setting of the seminary and especially the dormitory next door where we lived. This setting shielded us, and gradually permitted us to become acquainted with the city and what it had to offer. Seven of us who came from the provinces shared the same small dormitory room. We kept our belongings in lockers in the hallway. Five of us soon became a "five-some" who did almost everything together. We had a name for ourselves. In Hungary, a non-Jewish funeral cortege usually had five horses, so we named ourselves *Ötösfogat* like those five horses, and we snuck out of the dorm and enjoyed the city together.

Very quickly, I found out that *Shabbat* meant very little to my classmates. In my Seminary class of twelve, probably no more than three actually wanted to become Rabbis. The rest were more like me, unable to obtain a higher education elsewhere either because they were Jews, because they couldn't tolerate the anti-semitism, or because their families couldn't afford the tuition.

Everyone understood Yiddish but nobody spoke it. Everyone wanted to be educated in literary Hungarian so as to be able to deliver literate sermons. On Fridays they turned the lights on and off, hopped on the streetcars, spent money, went to the movies.

The first time this happened, it was a painful, painful experience that shattered my world. I practically cried that first Friday night because of this cataclysmic event. The real cataclysmic event, of course, was the fall of Poland, but my personal cataclysm was the collapse of my religion. I no longer believed what my parents believed, especially my mother.

I felt this way even though I had stopped fasting on Yom Kippur even before I left for Seminary. On Yom Kippur while everyone was in synagogue, Steve and I had slipped away and had something to eat at home. He had a cousin who was sure God would strike us dead, but of course nothing happened.

In Seminary, I was, however, very surprised to find that there was hardly a student who observed *kashrut*! The food that we got at the Seminary was fully kosher, but everyone also ate in restaurants where it was not.

The newness and hugeness of the city, the countless number of newspapers (compared to just a flimsy local one in Hajdúnánás), the libraries, museums, the many theaters, the Opera, the Symphony, the mountains around Buda offered us unprecedented opportunities for a broad, extracurricular education.

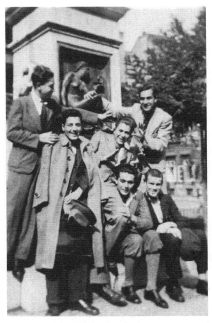

Rabbinical students on the town: Paul is seated, second from right.

There was even a brothel a block away from the Seminary, where, it was rumored, some of the older boys visited. I heard the rumors but did not know anyone who had been there. We took streetcars all over the city. I had relatives in Pest, my father's cousins, who invited me every Wednesday for the main meal. I also had other paternal relatives in Buda, where I took a weekly bath. Neither family kept kosher.

To take advantage of what Budapest had to offer, we needed money our parents could not provide. Luckily, we found jobs tutoring students in the different *gymnasia* as well as tutoring *bar mitzvah* boys. I even tutored a boy in English! I bought a Hungarian-English book of vocabulary and grammar, and made sure to keep a couple of lessons ahead of him. That was the way I learned my first sentences in English, the language that I was to speak for the rest of my life.

While all this tutoring took time away from my studies, there were months when I made more money at 16 and 17 in the city than my father was able to make as a middle-aged man in Hajdúnánás. I was able to help support my two younger brothers, who were in the Jewish Gymnasium in Debrecen.

Barely two months into my first year, I joined a study group with an upper-classman, Zvi Goldberg. He was 20, three years ahead of us, and had already decided that he wanted to become a psychoanalyst. He had a younger brother, Sanyi, in my class. Zvi invited him and five other first-year students to discuss psychoanalytic literature that he borrowed from the library. We met in Zvi's small, one-room apartment.

He taught in order to learn. He had a blackboard and we sat on the floor, willing to be his "guinea pigs." We read (in Hungarian) Freud's *Interpretation of Dreams*, Ferenczi's *Thalassa*, and Theodor Reik's *Ritual* — which explained, among other things, some cultural manifestations of Judaism for me — and I felt captivated. I realized that psychoanalysis was a way of thinking that went far deeper than graphology!

Even though I was interested in everything I was

learning in rabbinical school — the same curriculum as gymnasium plus Talmud, Bible and Hebrew language — all of it suddenly became secondary. I knew that, like Zvi, I wanted to become a psychoanalyst. These readings expanded my understanding of the world of the human psyche beyond my previous conceptions. I was then not yet drawn to the therapeutic implications of psychoanalysis. My interest, at first, was similar to that of a literary critic — in what we now call "applied psychoanalysis."

Freud's approach to dreams was an exciting way of getting to know my inner world and that of others. I soon learned that dreaming was a way we "naturally" communicate with ourselves but I had to learn what that communication from the depth of the psyche meant. How a dream was related to what you may have been thinking the day before but also how it was related to what you were striving for in your life.

The details of that first lecture have faded but I still remember how impressed I was by Zvi's intelligence, his teaching ability, his enthusiasm and his devotion.

Psychoanalysis soon supplanted my interest in graphology completely. When I first started wearing *tzitzit* as a boy in *cheder*, I never thought about what it meant. I only knew I was supposed to wear it. Reik's interpretation of Jewish rituals gave me an intriguing psychoanalytic explanation to what I had previously understood as a theology-based everyday practice. The psychoanalytic approach underscored much of what we learned and did at the Rabbinical Seminary. It enriched my outlook on life and made me reflect on the meaning of theologically-based "commandments" rather than just following them.

Ferenczi's *Thalassa* — later decried as pure fantasy —

made a lasting impression on me, even without my fully grasping its evolutionary meaning or significance, if any. At about the same time, I saw a short film about the drying-out of a huge lake in which a large number of small fish were "desperately" trying, head first, to bore themselves into the still wet mud, ostensibly trying to reach water. Just what Ferenczi imagined having happened in the course of evolution. He related this to his theory of sexuality in a way I no longer recall. This short film made the thesis of *Thalassa* plausible and real to me at that time. The more lasting impact of this was that I began to read Ferenczi's writings at the age of 16.

Zvi's reading group went on for a whole year, usually on Sunday afternoon, once or twice a month. But there was never enough time to read all I wanted to read. The demands of the Seminary and my tutoring schedule prevented further meetings after that first year. Tutoring allowed me to help support my brothers and send money home to my parents but curtailed my private reading. The question of having an actual analysis myself never presented itself to my mind even though some of Ferenczi's students were practicing in Budapest. I had no time and no money.

In Hungary in the early 1940s, you could either become a psychoanalyst by studying medicine or by going to university and studying psychology or philosophy. That was the direction Zvi chose. So I didn't, as a teenager, consider going to medical school. I was less interested in healing people than in the cultural and anthropological implications of psychoanalysis.

As I look back on my five years at the Seminary the ongoing "textual analysis" of the Bible and Talmud, without my full realization of it then, prepared me for "analytic thinking." The hermeneutic method became ingrained and imperceptibly a part of me. Freud's method of dream interpretation reminded me later of looking at single words and phrases in biblical and Talmudic texts to see what meaning was hidden in them or behind them and what associations could lead us to these hidden meanings.

I also received the full secular education I would later draw on in medical school. Every day from eight in the morning until about one o'clock, we studied a secular curriculum including physics and chemistry. In the afternoons I went from one pupil to the other, teaching science as well as language.

Paradoxically, as life around us became more and more difficult, we became more and more immersed in our own lives and studies, disavowing the probability that the dangerous conflagration would ultimately envelop all of us.

In December of 1941, I took the 12-hour train trip home to Hajdúnánás for Hanukah. My father had just been discharged from the forced labor battalion near Ungvár that he had served in since June. I was not alarmed by this. He had been an officer there, in charge of the group. Jews were still allowed to wear the uniforms of the Hungarian Army then — I had even been able to visit him. I saw no brutality, no barbed wire.

Now he was home again and seemed most interested in telling me that he had just visited his cousin Piri in Debrecen and that there was a nice young girl staying with her. My father had never made such a remark before, but I knew he didn't like the girl I was interested in at the time. He had always wanted me to meet his cousin Piri but I never went to see her, even though I had to change trains in Debrecen every time I traveled between Budapest and

Hajdúnánás. Now that he told me there was a young girl there, I went!

There was a snowstorm that evening. I arrived at about nine o'clock at night and stood knocking at the door for about ten minutes in the snow before a girl in a long robe let me in. People were fearful then, especially at night. I thought she was Piri, so I kissed her hand, as was the custom of the time.

Only after I got inside did I understand who was who. Piri was sitting inside, breast-feeding her six-month-old baby. Her husband had been taken to a labor battalion. Anna Brunn, who was 14 then, had opened the door for me. She had come from Szendrő to help her aunt and eventually attend Gymnasium.

I could stay only for about an hour because I had to catch the overnight train back to Budapest. As I walked to the train station, my hands froze because I had left my gloves behind. The train from Debrecen to Budapest took eight hours, so I had plenty of time to think about the girl. I was so impressed with Anna. She was three years younger than me, but much more interesting than the girl I was seeing in Hajdúnánás. We had a real conversation! She was so intelligent, poetic, vibrant and beautiful and she knew so much. I also loved her braids.

Although I was only 17, I already knew what I wanted. When I got to Budapest, I wrote a letter requesting that they send me my gloves and, if Anna wished, to please put a message for me in one of the fingers. She did so and I responded, and soon we were enjoying a regular correspondence.

In the summer, she went home to her family in Szendrő and I was able to ride my bicycle the close to 200 kilometers from our house to go see her. For the next two years, Anna spent the school year in Debrecen and I could visit her there.

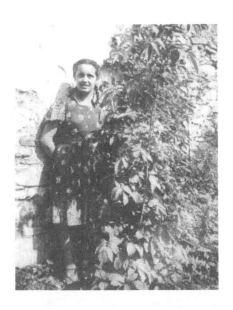

My father was very happy about this development and, until the spring of 1944, every time I changed trains in Debrecen on my way to or from Rabbinical Seminary, I stopped to see her. I also had spies to report on what she was doing: my two younger brothers attended school in Debrecen and reported to me if they saw that she was accompanied by another boy.

We exchanged dozens of letters.

Anna and I did not have the luxury of a prolonged transition from adolescence to adulthood. I realized that together we could make our dreams come true come hell or high water. We had a similar background, similar aspirations, and a Zionist orientation. We both knew that we would go to Palestine the moment that became possible, and create a life for ourselves together. For her 16th birthday I gave Anna a book of poetry by Charles Baudelaire titled *Toi et Moi* (*You and Me*) — that says it all.

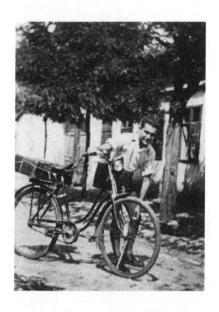

All this ended when the Germans invaded Hungary on March 19, 1944. I watched the soldiers march into Budapest, more and more of them, from the windows of our dormitory, which was connected by a short corridor to the seminary. Adolf Eichmann and his gang acted swiftly. They transformed the rabbinical school into a "Transit Camp" the same day they had arrived, and began to incarcerate the Jewish elite in the building prior to moving them on to the camp at Kistarcsa, a short distance from Budapest.

Our classrooms were emptied and straw pallets were put in for the important Budapest Jewish leaders to sleep on. But for some reason, they did not touch our dormitory. We, fifth-year students at the rabbinical school, were allowed to remain there and to see the prisoners. They asked us to take messages to their families in the city, which I and the others did. It didn't occur to me to run away. Nobody tried to escape. Nobody knew what would happen. The invasion brought an end to classes and it was impossible, under the circumstances, to focus on studying for exams. Usually students studied for their graduation exam for six months. Our teachers realized the difficulty of our situation, invited us to their homes, and gave us the exam questions there. Miraculously, we were able to graduate in May, under the Nazi Occupation, and had a ceremony attended by the Minister of Education, as was required by Hungarian law.

How was I picturing my future that May of 1944 just after I had turned 20? I knew for sure that I didn't want a pulpit and that I didn't want to stay in Hungary. I wanted to go to Palestine but I didn't see myself on a kibbutz. I wasn't yet thinking of medical school. Every reform Rabbi at that time in Hungary completed a Ph.D. and I thought I would too. I wasn't yet sure what I would study: perhaps the ancient languages and psychology. I wanted to become a psychoanalyst but didn't yet know what kind of psychology they taught at the university. I did not like armchair theorizing and wanted to have direct analytic contact with patients to get at empirical data that would give me a firmer platform.

We were, in May of 1944, totally unaware of the Nazis' industrialized extermination program that was underway as we were taking our final exams in Budapest. I would not learn about the extermination camps for another six months.

In May, shortly after my graduation, I was conscripted, along with my father and several thousand Jewish men for forced labor. By that time, we knew something about labor battalions but nothing about death camps. Some upper-classmen had already been sent to perform forced labor. Others were living in Budapest on false papers. One student obtained false papers and went around the city dressed as a Protestant minister.

I, like my classmates, had a certificate from the Ministry of Interior, that as a rabbinical student I was exempt from military or paramilitary service. I expected to be promptly released on arrival at the collection center, and planned to procure false "Aryan papers," and hide under that new identity for the remainder of the war. But the general to whom I had to submit my certificate simply tore it up and said "such things no longer count." So, that escape route was closed.

I was assigned, along with my friend and fellow rabbinical student Gyuri Auspitz, to battalion 101/95 and an uncertain future. At the time, I was most upset at having to leave Budapest and my younger sister Judit.

Judit had left the Hajdúnánás Gymnasium after her fourth year and followed me to Budapest in 1942. She loved to dance and under other circumstances would have gone to gymnasium for eight years. As it was, she came to Budapest to pursue training as a dental technician. The idea was to have a skill with which to support herself. Her workplace was located a short walk from where I lived and we were in close contact, which was emotionally supportive to us both. We went to the movies together. Sometimes on Friday nights, she and her eleven roommates made *erev Shabbat* dinner. After the rabbinical school student who officiated on Friday nights went into forced labor, I took over his duties and I officiated at a kind of service. When I said good-bye to her in 1944, neither of us could imagine that it was final — that we would never see each other again.

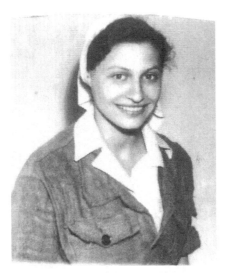

Judit Ornstein at about the age of 16

THREE ~ 1944

In early June 1944, Battalion 101/95 was ordered to appear in Jászberény military headquarters; then we were dispatched to Várpalota — south of Budapest, where we were to build an airport runway. It was there that I received two postcards, one from Anna, (with whom by now I was madly in love), telling me that they were herded into a ghetto in their village of Szendrő and would be deported within days; and one from my brother Zoli, who threw his postcard from a cattle wagon, saying that he, our mother and my other two brothers were taken from the ghetto in Hajdúnánás to an unknown destination. My father, I knew, was in a forced labor battalion. This was the last mail I received about them.

The news was demoralizing. Though others received similar messages about deportation, we were not sure what they meant. We lulled ourselves into believing that our situation was different, that we were needed for important work for the armed forces and the German-Hungarian war effort and therefore protected. This was a realistic assumption at the time but turned out to be a near-delusional belief.

In July, we were transferred out of Hungary and across the Carpathian Mountains to the Eastern Front. We made camp between Stanislau and Kolomea, (then Poland, now the Ukraine) to work for the Hungarian army facing the Russians who appeared to be preparing an attack.

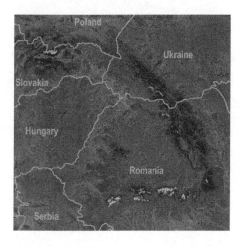

Sporadic *katyusha* rockets were fired in our direction as we were digging ditches to prepare a defensive line for the Hungarian and German armies against the advancing Russians. This was a ridiculously ineffective undertaking.

We soon created a new five-some, Gyuri and I and three other schoolmates: Öcsi, Böci and Béla. As a group we protected each other, sharing food and rations. Since none of us smoked, we could barter our very valuable cigarettes for bread. We dealt with important issues democratically — we voted, especially when it came to decisions about survival strategies.

Our emotional state was paradoxical: we wanted the Russians to advance against the Germans, though we could easily become their first victims. We had no sympathy for our Hungarian "superiors"; they deserved none.

Early on a Sunday morning in September of 1944, we were digging trenches again when a barrage of *katyusha* fire began. The German army had left the day before, leaving the Hungarians to cover them as they retreated. By mid-morning, the Hungarian soldiers also began to retreat, while threatening to shoot us, if we did not continue digging. After a short while, we too began to retreat, since the *katyushas* were landing dangerously close.

Two-hundred yards from the trenches, I suddenly realized that I left my jacket behind. Gyuri told me to leave it behind, afraid that the rockets would hit me. But I had photographs of Anna and my family in the pocket of that jacket and they were my talisman.

Gyuri returned with me to retrieve my jacket. We then crawled back on our bellies. In the pandemonium, everyone ran in whatever direction he could toward the Carpathian mountains, toward Hungary.

At one point, we reached a small forest and a group of about 20 to 25 members of our battalion got into a discussion of whether we should try to remain behind and get over to the Russian side. They imagined that by telling the Russians that we were Jews, we would be given special privileges and might even be assigned to supervise the German and Hungarian prisoners of war. Gyuri and I thought that was wishful thinking. Our five-some decided that in such a life-and-death matter we should not expect each other to abide by a majority decision but should allow everyone to choose his own fate.

Three in the group decided to remain behind and try to get to the Russians. Gyuri and I decided to keep running. We thought — mistakenly as it turned out — that we were only about 20 kilometers from the Carpathian Mountains and we hoped to cross back into Hungarian territory, where we knew the language. Gyuri and I helped those who chose to wait for the Russians to dig a hiding place in the ground and cover it with tree branches for protection against detection by the Hungarian military police. We then gave them some of our clothes and food and quickly moved on, fearing for their lives.

Gyuri and I turned out to be correct. The Jewish prisoners in Russia did not receive special treatment because they were Jews. They were treated like the Hungarian Nazis and the SS prisoners. Many died in Siberia, but Öcsi, Böci and Béla returned after five years of captivity to Budapest. Béla became a surgeon; the other two had many ailments and never attained their pre-war potential.

Gyuri and I spent the twenty-four hours after we left them in the swarm of Hungarian soldiers and forced laborers marching toward the Carpathian Mountains in retreat from the Russian Army. At day-break we reached a plateau, still in Polish territory, where camp commanders began to reassemble survivors of their battalions. Ours regrouped.

As we continued to march, we realized that we were actually *60* — not 20 — kilometers away from the border. Had we known that, Gyuri and I would have dug ourselves into the hole with the others and risked the consequences.

After another two days of marching, our battalion stopped in a clearing in the middle of a beautiful mountain-pass that connected Poland with Hungary. I would have enjoyed being there under other circumstances, but being on the front line was stressful and extremely dangerous.

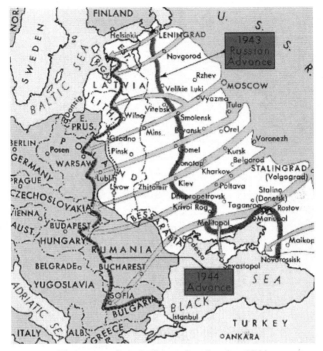

The eastern front in September-October 1944

The hard work, hunger, corporal punishment and other kinds of mistreatment were not the main traumata inflicted on us in this setting. What was more difficult to endure were the deliberately degrading and humiliating verbal and physical attacks by our Hungarian guards, along with the expectation that we perform efficiently despite them. Not having any news of our families' fate and whereabouts added a sense of foreboding to our daily existence. Our own fate was also highly uncertain.

At one point, we worked on a mountainside, cutting trees and hauling the logs to create a thoroughfare for the retreating German and Hungarian tanks, and other military vehicles. Under optimal circumstances each log would have required ten to twelve men. At times, our Hungarian guards deliberately assigned fewer conscripts than needed. To add insult to injury, they often specifically solicited lawyers or academics for such work, pretending that they were needed for desk jobs. Those men who hoped to get a better assignment for the day were tricked into doing the hardest or the most demeaning tasks. Then our guards screamed obscenities and anti-semitic slogans at them, here and there underscoring their contempt and hatred with beatings.

Some men could not survive this kind of abuse. Some disappeared during the retreat from the Russians; I don't know if they died or managed to escape and survive. The treatment was brutal and, obviously, unfair. I remember one man who took it particularly hard; he didn't feel Jewish; he believed he was there by mistake. My friend Gyuri lost his will to live for a time. I did not. I felt as long as we were headed towards Hungary, there was hope. Somehow I remained optimistic; I always thought that I would find some way to get home.

September, however, is windy, cold and rainy in the Carpathian Mountains. Because we had given some of our clothes away and discarded others to lighten our backpacks, I began to worry that I would freeze to death. I was obsessed with the idea of getting back to Hungary, where at least I could speak the language. One of my ideas to escape was to pretend I was ill. I would need a kind of medical care that the battalion physician could not provide, necessitating my being sent to the military infirmary and field hospital. I also decided that I could only survive if I would be sent to a hospital *inside* Hungary, where I could escape to a farm and have a farmer's daughter fall in love with me and hide me until the Russians arrived. A bold and naïve plan, but I became obsessed with it as my only salvation.

Pretending to be ill carried the risk that if the Hungarian military physician found me healthy, there was a punishment: no food for the next twenty-four hours, or a worse work assignment. I needed to have some sort of illness that required surgery, but what sort? I settled on appendicitis. I had no medical knowledge at the time but questioned people who did. Appendicitis seemed to be the answer. I talked with people whose appendix had been removed, then I asked to be sent to the infirmary. On examination, I was diagnosed as having a bladder infection and given medications which I promptly discarded. I made several "follow-up" trips and learned a great deal about how the infirmary worked and what I needed to do to succeed in my plan.

Meanwhile, another decimated Jewish forced labor battalion arrived to join ours. There was a physician among them whom I consulted about my plan. He told me that if I had appendicitis, I had to have a fever. On my next visit to the infirmary, when I was given a thermometer and asked to sit outside the examining room until called in again, I rubbed the thermometer between my fingers and raised the mercury to a level that indicated fever. The examining physician and a higher-ranking consultant decided that I had to be operated on the next morning. I was given a badge to wear. It had on it the diagnosis of "acute appendicitis" and the time of my scheduled operation the next morning: 9:00 AM.

For the first time since I left Budapest, I became immensely frightened. I suddenly thought of many things I had not considered before. I hadn't thought to ask whether the surgeon would recognize that my appendix was not infected — that's how naïve I was! He might become enraged and not even close me up but leave me to die! How long would the recovery take? Would the Russians attack while I was still convalescing and capture me? These fears kept me awake all night.

Early in the morning we heard bombardment from a distance. All patients waiting for operations were lined up to be seen by the Chief of the field hospital and his entourage. Each of us was asked just one question: "Could you walk a few kilometers?" I broke out in a sweat, frightened that if I said yes, it might betray me, but if I said no, I might not be evacuated.

When my turn came, I contorted my face and said: "Y-e-s, I w-ill try" conveying my pain, but readiness to walk if I had to. It worked. As we were leaving, a convoy of empty trucks was coming from the front line on their way to Hungary to bring back needed ammunition. The hospital authorities asked them to take us across the border to the first Red Cross station in Hungarian territory.

I got on the truck. At the first Red Cross station, a few people were taken off for urgent care but I was sent on. It happened a second time. I was happy to be back inside Hungary, but began to worry: how long could I reasonably be suffering from acute appendicitis and not pass out? It was in the middle of the night when we arrived at the third or fourth Red Cross station. A women physician examined me, the gentlest and kindest military doctor I had yet encountered. She asked me whether I was able to hold on until we reached a hospital where they could operate. Gentle and kind she was, but knowledgeable she was not! I was overjoyed to be getting deeper into Hungary. I could now speak to people and hope to implement my plans for escape.

I must have been *en route* for two or three days. It was September 26, 1944, Yom Kippur eve, when I arrived at a sprawling, makeshift hospital, housing several thousand forced laborers returning from various parts of the Russian front.

I knew more about appendicitis now, after having been repeatedly examined. I could ask questions I never thought of before and this comforted and calmed me and gave me courage. In this place, however, the military surgeons were thorough and skillful. Mine kept talking to me while he examined my belly, distracting me, so that I failed to react to the "pain." He astutely diagnosed me as a "*simulant*" and put on the upper right-hand edge of my discharge paper "back to hard labor."

The next day, ten of us Jews, in custody of four Hungarian soldiers, were sent by train back toward the Carpathians. The guards held our discharge papers but, luckily, some members of our group still had money. They bought some alcohol and offered it to the guards, who promptly got drunk and fell asleep. We then stole our discharge papers from the sleeping soldiers and got off the train.

What to do now? We decided to continue to our destination and insist that we had been discharged, unguarded. The proof was that we had our papers. Telephones were no longer working reliably, nothing could be verified. I was still terrified, but feeling lucky to have escaped without an operation for my non-existent appendicitis. I continued to imagine that a farmer's daughter would fall in love with me and hide me. How a farmer's daughter, in the notoriously anti-semitic Hungarian countryside of 1944, could fall in love with a fugitive Jew was never allowed to enter my consciousness.

It was late in the evening, when our train arrived at the last station on the Hungarian side of the border. The military dispatcher's office would not be open till the next morning. As the night wore on my anxiety mounted, until I came up with the idea of falsifying one digit in the number of my unit on my papers. Knowing that 101/96 was in Budapest, I decided to change 101/95 into 101/96 — that would do the trick. I was certain that the dispatcher would not find the new number on his map, because it was out of range. I borrowed a pen from a friendly-looking soldier and in the dim light of the toilet, I changed the number. Relieved and hopeful, I could now fall asleep sitting in the waiting room of the train station.

Near panic gripped me at dawn, when I realized in the daylight that my number 6 was in a different color ink than the rest of the numbers. Any attentive dispatcher could have recognized that. But by the time the office opened, I had my wits available to me again.

At the dispatchers' table, four soldiers stood behind the counter, a huge map on the wall behind them, with small flags marking the location of every military and forced labor unit in the region — on the Russian front and Northeastern Hungary. A single line formed in front of each soldier. Three of them held on to the marching papers handed to them as they searched for the location. The fourth soldier looked at the number, returned the papers and searched the map. I quickly joined that line.

As I anticipated, he could not find 101/96. That unit was in Budapest, out of the range of his map. When he apologetically directed me back inland, I was overjoyed. Here was my opportunity to walk *legally* in the countryside, speak my language, have my papers stamped, get food every 24 hours, and search for a farm where I might find temporary work and lodging, and a farmer's daughter. A number of my efforts failed. I was repeatedly turned away; some farmers did so with abusive threats. But one evening, I was able to find work helping with the harvest of corn. There was no daughter but friendly farmers. I spent the night in their barn and left very early, not knowing what their attitude might be in the morning.

I felt encouraged by getting still deeper into Hungary and arrived by train at Sátoraljaújhely on October 15. There, the Military Police emptied the train and we were taken to an old army garrison where we heard Admiral Horthy's radio message abrogating the treaty with Germany and declaring neutrality. By evening, we found out that he had been immediately arrested, deported to Germany, and the new Hungarian Nazi Government was now trying to complete what Eichmann began.

Horthy had ordered all Hungarian troops back to Hungary. The Hungarian soldiers now rounded us up and shipped us by train to Miskolc (about 150 kilometers northeast of Budapest), where we were ordered to march toward the Austrian border. The trip took nearly two weeks; we slept in fields and in the forests. As we passed near Budapest, I was able to sneak onto a truck filled with forced laborers from Szendrő, Anna's hometown. One of them recognized me and I was able to make my way back to the city and reach the home of my father's cousins in Pest.

It was a Sunday, a day when Hungarians dressed up to go to church. I was filthy, unshaven for weeks, wearing rags. I was only able to ride the streetcar to the center of the city because a total stranger, a Jew living with false papers in Budapest, recognized my situation and bought me a ticket. He also told me that some neutral countries such as Sweden and Switzerland had organized "safe houses" for Jews under the aegis of their embassies and that there were over two thousand Jews being protected in the "glass house," a former glass factory in Pest.

Although Hungarian authorities had already deported some 440,000 Jews who lived outside Budapest to extermination camps, primarily to Auschwitz, most of the Budapest Jewish community was still alive. Some Jews, such as my relatives, were still living in their own homes. These were called "yellow star" houses, specially marked and also protected by the neutral countries. Their occupants could only go out between ten and twelve in the morning. I actually arrived later than that. There was a Hungarian soldier at the entrance, talking to the janitor's son and he should not have allowed me to enter. But the janitor's son recognized me from my weekly visits during rabbinical school and told him that I lived there.

My relatives were astonished and very happy to see me. They knew I had been taken to forced labor somewhere on the Ukrainian front and thought I had died. My welcome, however, was postponed until I could take a bath — I was very dirty and covered with lice. It was the first time I had been able to wash in hot water in almost six months. They threw out all my clothing and gave me replacements, probably their son's clothes. Then they prepared a meal and we talked.

I didn't ask them what they knew about my father, my mother, and my brothers because I knew they couldn't know anything that was going on outside of Budapest. But

I immediately asked about my sister Judit who, when I left Budapest a few months earlier, was working as a dental technician. They seemed evasive. All they were able to tell me was that Judit had been expected to come to their house for dinner the evening before Yom Kippur and had not arrived. Maybe, they said, "Judit went west." I was so exhausted that I accepted what they said for the moment, went to their son's bed next to the kitchen, and went to sleep.

First thing the next morning, I walked to the building where Judit lived. When I got there, I saw that half the building no longer existed: it had been destroyed by a bomb. I had already suspected the worst when my relatives told me that she must have gone "west." The man in charge of the building had a list of the inhabitants, and he confirmed that my sister had been among those killed.

When we were children, Judit was always teasing me. In Budapest, we had a very loving relationship. She was my only sister. For some reason, we never went out alone in the city. She was always with her girlfriends. We only met when she came to the Seminary not far from where she worked and called up to the window of my dormitory. Not until long after the war was over, was I able to visit her grave.

Many years later, Anna received a letter from a woman in Israel. This woman explained, in Hungarian, that she had lived with Judit Ornstein in the dormitory. When the bombing had begun, a teacher got all the girls out of the building. Judit had a sore leg at the time and couldn't run out with them. The teacher went back in to get her and both were killed. Along with the letter was a copy of a photo she had retrieved from the rubble.

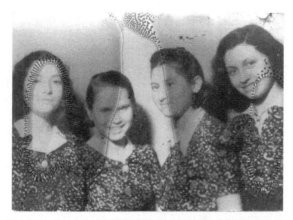

Photo retrieved from the bombed out building, Judit at right.

That Monday in 1944, I decided to go to the glass house that the man who bought me a streetcar ticket had told me was under the protection of the Swiss Embassy. I had never heard of this former glass factory when I was a student. Now there were over 2,000 Jews taking refuge there and in the adjoining houses, among them members of the Zionist underground. I felt sure I would find some of my old schoolmates there.

When I arrived, there were hundreds of people in the street, shouting and demanding papers, anything to help them get out of the country.

It was difficult to hear anything at all in that noise, but I finally heard someone shouting my name and noticed friends of mine motioning me to come to an open window and shouting to me.

A couple of people pulled me up off the street and through that window into the building.

Inside it was very crowded. People were sleeping so close together that at time you couldn't turn over at night. There I found many friends and acquaintances. There was some food brought into the building for the noon meal.

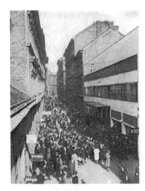

People gathered before the glass house

I spent November and part of December in the glass house, stupidly daring. I would go in and out to visit my relatives and work for the Zionist underground. Twelve of us went out every day between ten and twelve to help the people who were in safe houses. We felt protected. Many of my friends were there and I started talking with one of them, Kala Feldman, about going to Palestine as soon as we could.

The siege of Budapest by the Red Army began in December 1944 and lasted until mid-February 1945. During that time, the city was in chaos, with enormous destruction, including the blowing up of all the bridges across the Danube by the Germans.

Before the siege was over we heard that the Russians

had consolidated their forces at Debrecen, on the way to Hajdúnánás, so one night Kala, who was from Debrecen, and I decided to take a chance and leave. Today, by car, it takes a little over two hours to drive the highway from Budapest to Debrecen. It took us much longer because we walked, were arrested by Russian soldiers and once again forced to work. Once again, I planned an escape and succeeded. Kala and I then walked across the Tisza river over a bridge that was almost completely destroyed. But we managed to get to the other side, and then were able to take a train to our respective homes.

When I finally reached Hajdúnánás, it was late at night in February. There were strangers living in my home. I found an abandoned house and went to sleep there. When I woke up, I walked to the synagogue. It was also occupied by strangers. No one knew anything about what had happened to the members of my family. No one could find out anything. There was no telephone. No radio. Everything was hearsay. I heard that my friend Steve Hornstein had come back and was living about half a mile from the train station.

Steve could take me in. He had gotten back to Hajdúnánás a month before and had a room with a Christian family with a sofa in his room in addition to his bed. Steve and I looked much the same as before the war. Although a cataclysm had occurred, not so much time had passed — only seven months. He told me about his experience in forced labor inside Hungary, on the western side of the Danube. It hadn't been so bad. He had been very lucky.

Now all he wanted was to start medical school in Debrecen as soon as possible. He wasn't a Zionist. He had an idea that he had a role to play in Hungary. He changed his name to a Hungarian name. I didn't argue with him; I figured that was his issue. By that time, I was thinking that I should go to medical school too but not in Hungary. At that point, I thought: everything here is in ruins. I'm going to try to go to medical school in Palestine with Kala. When my family gets back, they will follow me. I had made sure with my Budapest friends that they would get in touch with me if they heard anything about Anna or my family. I now told Steve that I would write when I got to Palestine.

Kala and I took a train to Bucharest en route, we thought, to Palestine. When we got there, we met Hungarian Zionists waiting and found enough to eat, but no way to get to Palestine. Since neither of us wanted to return to Hungary, we began our medical studies at the Hungarian University's Medical School in Cluj (Klausenburg) in Transylvania. Cluj had a pre-war Jewish community to which Jews were returning after the war. We had very little money but the American Joint Jewish Committee was there to help us and we also found lodging. There I was able to contact my one relative in America, the sister of my mother who had left Hajdúnánás in the 1920s and lived in Easton, Pennsylvania. They sent me packages.

That February of 1944, as I began studying chemistry in Cluj, I was still bent on becoming a psychoanalyst, but with psychoanalysis so linguistically rooted, I thought: what will I do if I end up in a jungle of South America? I was looking to the future and thought that, as an immigrant, I could practice medicine anywhere. I didn't know at the time that you had to have a license, or you won't be allowed to practice.

So I thought it would be worthwhile to suffer through medical school but it turned out to be no suffering at all! I even liked anatomy. I got to know the brain and to be comfortable with patients suffering from psychosomatic problems. I buried myself in my studies until, in August of 1945, my friends at the Jewish Committee's Receiving and Debriefing Center in Budapest notified me that my father and Anna had been seen alive after liberation by some of the returnees. As it happened, Anna returned from Auschwitz with her mother, and my father returned from Mauthausen during the same week.

I received a telegram about their arrival and rushed to Budapest. That meant sneaking onto a freight train and hoping for the best — there were not too many directions a train could travel: from Cluj to Debrecen; from there mainly in the direction of Pest, with all sorts of interim stops. The trip lasted two to three days, in a wagon without a roof, a trip which, under ordinary circumstances, would take slightly more than half a day.

I went to see Anna first. She was asleep when I entered her aunt's apartment, where she and her mother had found temporary shelter. I stood at her bedside, trembling. By then we all knew what "deportation" meant and how few people remained alive. When Anna woke up, we fell into each other's arms and our tears began to flow, joy and pain mixed, we could barely let go of each other.

Then I rushed to meet my father at his cousin's apartment. He was skin and bones after months in Gunskirchen (one of many outer camps of Mauthausen). He was in deep despair over the death of my sister Judit, his only daughter. His reaction to seeing me revived his spirits — now there were reasons again to go on living, he said — and he began to chastise me lovingly for having gone to see Anna first.

I persuaded both Anna and my father to join me in Cluj,

while I prepared for my examinations. There was ample food in Cluj, while there was very little of it in Budapest; and there Anna and my father could be placed in a specially prepared hostel for returnees for two to four weeks. The three of us smuggled ourselves into another freight train and managed to successfully arrive in Cluj.

Over a period of several weeks, Anna told me about her concentration camp experiences and I told her about mine in the forced labor battalion. But soon, planning for our future took center stage. Anna focused on completing her interrupted schooling.

Kala and I completed our exams in physics and chemistry. Then we were kicked out and forced to return to Budapest, since we were not Romanian citizens. At the end of the summer of 1945, my father, Anna and I returned to Budapest on another freight train.

My father returned to Hajdúnánás and opened an office for book-keeping and tax-related services. Anna studied for her "matura-certificate" and I started my second year of medical school in Budapest. I was hoping to finish medical school there and Anna was planning to start her medical studies after her "matura." Then we would leave the country for Palestine. But I became increasingly worried by the political situation in Hungary.

The results of the first democratic election in November 1945 were alarming. Every morning we read the papers.

The Hungarian Communist Party received less than 20 percent of the vote; the Independent Smallholders' Party won 57 percent of the vote. But the Soviet commander in Hungary refused to allow the Smallholders' Party to form a government. Instead, he established a coalition government with the Communists holding some of the key posts. The

Kingdom of Hungary was formally abolished on February 1, 1946, and replaced by the Republic of Hungary.

I felt certain that the Hungarian Communists, with the help of the Russians, would take over and that we would all be stuck in Hungary.

My Pest relatives did not wish to leave. They were jewelers who had established their business in Budapest. But they did business in Switzerland, and had connections to the Swiss Consulate. Somehow they were able to arrange the promise of a scholarship for Anna and me to study medicine in Switzerland. This would have been ideal, but the Consulate made the visa contingent on a scholarship, and the scholarship agency made the scholarship contingent on a visa. The impasse could not be overcome. We decided to leave Hungary and then try to get visas through the Swiss Consulate in Vienna.

By then, Steve Hornstein had changed his mind about becoming Hungarian and his brother Karl also wanted to leave with us. They never told me why and I didn't ask.

Emotionally it was not difficult for me to leave Hungary — I was ready for it already when I set out for Bucharest, but it was difficult for Anna to leave her mother behind. Sophie was 48 then and Anna was her only surviving child. Her two sons, ages 20 and 22, did not return from forced labor. In addition, she had very meaningful and interesting work running the Rákosszentmihály orphanage, an orphanage for Jewish children whose parents had been murdered by the Nazis. Sophie did not want to join us because she loved her work and also for fear that she might become dependent on us. My father, on the other hand, was sure he wanted to emigrate — at the age of 50! — to Palestine. He thought we would follow him there.

Anna and I were married in the garden of the orphanage on March 13, 1946. A few weeks later, we were smuggled across the border with my father in a car by the commanding officer of the Russian Border Guards to the American sector of Vienna. In the car with me were Anna, my father, my friend Steve, and his brother Karl.

We had $100, accumulated from gifts from relatives in the U.S. and from wedding presents and used it to pay for the illegal trip. The Russian officer took $30 from each of us for the ride. We arrived with almost no money at the Rothschild Hospital, the Viennese transit camp for Jewish refugees from the East.

We were there for six weeks. When we presented ourselves to the Swiss Consulate, they asked for our passports and when we told them that we had none, their response was simple and final: without passports we could not get entry permits to study in Switzerland. That killed our wonderful plan.

We had two choices then. One was to go to a Displaced Persons (DP) camp in Italy and try to study medicine at a university there, but we were afraid that we wouldn't be able to learn Italian quickly or well enough. The second choice was to go to a DP camp in Germany where we anticipated less difficulty with the language and where the universities were better. We were so future-oriented that the place we would study mattered less to us than the education we wanted. Even though it was Germany, we knew there was a Jewish Student Union there and that we were going to the U.S. occupied zone. The "*bricha*" — the Jewish underground — transported us along with many other refugees across the Russian zone of Austria, via Salzburg, to the closest village across the border on the German side: the village of Ainring.

To have escaped to the West, gave us the unexpected opportunity to travel, something we had never done before. I can't say that, at the time, we mastered our rage and grief. We postponed dealing with them. In retrospect, I can see that we were numb in a certain way, more than we realized then. The fact that Anna and I met again brought us back to life together. I have often thought that the so-called "survival guilt" is in many ways a figment of the imagination of psychoanalysts who escaped from Europe on time. We did not suffer from "survival guilt." In spite of everything, we were able to enjoy life.

Within a couple of weeks, that summer of 1946, we were settled in the DP camp of Deggendorf, in the U.S. Occupied Zone of Bavaria, Germany.

FOUR ~ Germany

Steve and I were admitted to medical school in Munich two hours away from the camp by train. Steve had by then met Lusia Schwarzwald, a young Polish Jew from Lvov, Poland whom he had met on the train. I thought he had been very smart to start up a conversation with her. She was good-looking, thoughtful and if anything more intelligent than my friend! Although she had been at music conservatory in Vienna, she now joined Anna at UNRRA (United Nations Relief and Rehabilitation Administration) University — a makeshift University for the refugees who were not eligible to enter the German Universities.

Although we were very happy to have left Hungary and to be living and studying in the U.S. zone, Munich was an unpleasant place in 1946. Many of the houses and streets were destroyed. It had been severely bombed during the war. Life was difficult. Anna and I lived in one small cramped and inadequate room with a small bed — and Steve Hornstein and I soon set out to find another medical school. We visited Frankfurt and Heidelberg. It was easy to be admitted in Frankfurt, but Heidelberg, which was more difficult, was our first choice.

Heidelberg was a beautiful medieval town of about 100,000 on the Neckar River. The university, founded in 1378, was one of the oldest in Europe. The town had

69

escaped all bombing during the war and had now been made the European headquarters of the U.S. Army.

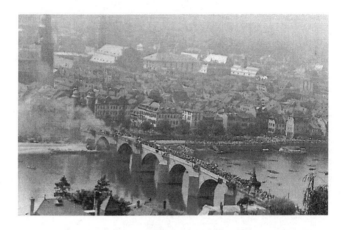

Admission for foreign students was administered by the UNRRA and only a limited number were admitted. A Canadian Jewish female officer was in charge. We spent a whole day trying to persuade her — in our broken German, since we did not yet speak English — that we should be allowed to study in Heidelberg. After a day of struggle she finally promised Steve and me that if we completed our "Physikum" with good grades in Munich, we would be admitted for the clinical years at the University of Heidelberg. We were too embarrassed to ask her to give us her promise in writing.

Steve and I spent the academic year of 1946-1947 in Munich studying Zoology, Botany, Anatomy, Physiology (and related subjects) for the Physikum; on weekends we would return to Deggendorf, where my father worked for the UNRRA as a book-keeper. He was able to help us supplement our rations, which were meager in post-war Germany.

We were all excellent students and, one year later, Steve and I returned to Heidelberg and proudly presented our credentials to the Canadian International Relief Organization gate-keeper, reminding her of the promise she made to us the previous year. At first she insisted that that she did not recognize us and that she did not recall any such promise. But when we reminded her of our day-long effort at persuading her to accept us, she finally accompanied us to the "Questura," the office where we had to register for admission.

That done, we returned with her to her office. She could not understand why we were following her back. "We have wives," we said. Our wives had completed one year of study in Munich and we wanted them to continue their medical studies in Heidelberg. After a year as students in Germany, we now spoke the language fluently and could calmly argue our case. She turned to us with visible anger: "Why didn't you tell me last year?"

"Had we done so," we replied, "you would not have admitted us either." She burst out laughing and said: "OK, send your wives to see me."

They too, were admitted to study in Heidelberg in 1947.

That June, we left the Deggendorf DP camp and my father behind. He had never deviated from his plan to make *aliya* and was finally able to emigrate to the one-year-old State of Israel in 1949. I thought that we would pursue our medical education in Heidelberg and eventually join him there.

Meanwhile, Anna and I, Steve and Lusia all moved to Heidelberg. The university had been thoroughly Nazi in the

1930s, the site of Nazi book burnings and eugenics experiments. Members of its Jewish and anti-Nazi faculty had been fired. Some had emigrated, some were deported, at least two were murdered. Closed when the war ended, it was reopened in January of 1946 through the efforts of philosopher Karl Jaspers and surgeon Karl Heinrich Bauer. Now, Heidelberg University was undergoing a de-Nazification program.

It was in this atmosphere that it and other major German universities such as Tübingen were accepting applications both from returning German soldiers and from refugee Jews like ourselves. We were no longer Hungarians. We were stateless; citizens of no country; we held no passports.

In his book *Remember: My Stories of Survival and Beyond*, Marcel Tuchman, one of the first Jewish students we met there, describes Heidelberg at the end of 1945 as "teeming with the American military presence. GIs in jeeps and on foot in their slick Eisenhower jackets were cheerful, friendly and informal, and were seen everywhere.

The loudspeakers near military installations in the city blared the familiar tunes of the Glenn Miller Orchestra — *Chattanooga Choo-Choo* and *Moonlight Serenade* — and the voice of Rosemary Clooney crooned the rhythmic *Come on to My House* from the American Forces network. The festive atmosphere was infectious.

We strongly identified with our liberators, feeling secure, free, and jolly for the first time in years. The tragic experiences of the recent past were curiously submerged, at least for that magic moment in history, as we were rapt with resurrection fantasy."

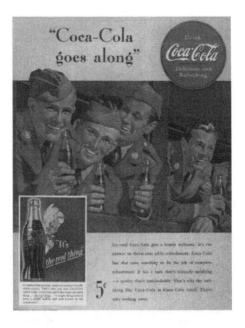

Marcel Tuchman had been one of the first Jewish medical students to arrive in Heidelberg. He was from Przemyśl, Poland, had survived the war as a slave laborer in Auschwitz, and arrived from the DP camp at Bergen-Belsen. "The Germans in town kept a low profile," he wrote. "They were quiet in defeat, respectful and obsequious, even servile when confronted by the Americans. With regard to us, they repressed their true inner feelings of resentment and shame in defeat. None of the Germans admitted they had known about the atrocities that had been committed.

"When I looked around the classroom, what held my attention was that many young men who had returned to the university to continue their studies, which had been interrupted by the war, still wore parts of their military uniform — the military boots and breeches. It now seems a trivial detail, but to one with my experience it provoked an uneasy reaction."

We got to Heidelberg almost two years after Marcel Tuchman and the atmosphere was quieter. But it was still clear that the Americans were very much in charge. We knew that there were trials of Nazis going on. The incident that I remember best with the American Army involved a pair of khaki pants. Unbeknownst to us, there was a regulation at the time that no one but members of the American forces could wear them. I had a cousin from Pennsylvania who was serving in the military in Europe and he gave me a pair of his pants. One day I was standing on the steps of a building with my father who was visiting. A pair of MPs on a motorcycle passed me, then turned around and arrested me! They took me immediately to HQ and a few minutes later to jail, where I spent a few hours. I was stripped and given different clothing. I was angry at them so I tore off some pieces of the pants as a souvenir. Marcel Tuchman, who had many connections by then, got me out.

Our most influential friend in Heidelberg was a German — a Lutheran pastor, Pfarrer Hermann Ludwig Maas. Maas was born in 1877. In 1903, he had begun working as a Protestant minister in Baden and became friendly with Zionist Jews there. He had heard Theodor Herzl speak at the Sixth Zionist Congress in Basel. He spoke fluent Hebrew and displayed both a *mezuzah* and a cross in his home. On Rosh Hashana and Yom Kippur he came to *daven* at our services and prayed with a *tallis* over his head (I had stopped praying a long time before but I still attended services, because I enjoyed the readings I remembered from my childhood without worrying about God). Pfarrer Maas came to like my mother-in-law Sophie very much, and continued to visit her after Anna and I left for the United States and she remained in Heidelberg.

Like Protestant theologians Dietrich Bonhoeffer and Martin Niemöller, Pfarrer Maas had been a rare advocate for Jews under Nazism. He had helped many Jews leave Germany. In 1943, the Nazis had forced him out of office and in 1944, he had himself been deported to a work camp. In 1950, Maas was the first non-Jewish German to be officially invited to the newly formed state of Israel. On July 28, 1964, Yad Vashem recognized him as one of the Righteous Among the Nations.

Pfarrer Maas was of course an exception. We all rented rooms or apartments from German families with whom our relations ranged from strained to polite. The first place we stayed, the woman's husband was still a German war prisoner; she didn't want us to use her kitchen. In another place, the owners were much nicer and pretended to be happy we were there. I heard them thanking the placement agency for sending us but I didn't believe them. They had two daughters and a son and Anna often had conversations with them in the kitchen. I rarely went out of my room. After two years, my mother-in-law arrived and we moved in with the widow of a former professor of psychology. Here, the three of us shared two rooms. Frau Muckle genuinely welcomed us. We had free access to her well-stocked library. She gave us two rooms. She and her husband had not been Nazis; they had been Social Democrats and friends of Pfarrer Maas.

We knew that our professors were former Nazis, but our relationship with them was never personal as it often is in the United States. Lectures were formal, given in large lecture halls. None of the Jewish students socialized with our German classmates either. We sat together at lectures. We studied together, even shared the same corpses for dissections. Instead of eating at the university *Mensa* with the other students, we ate our main meal of the day together at the Jewish Student Union. Our isolation from the German students and the knowledge that we were in Germany for a definite purpose and *only* in transition to permanent homes in Israel or the United States or some other Western country, made it psychologically possible for us to live and study there.

The packages we all received from relatives in the United States supplemented our German rations. My aunt in Easton, Pennsylvania sent packages of clothing; Anna had an uncle in New York who sent packages of coffee and cigarettes. As in the labor battalion, cigarettes were the best currency. And we did not smoke!! We sold the cigarettes and the clothing that did not fit us on the black market and, with the money, bought books, our own microscope, went to the movies, and bought food that we shared with our friends at the Jewish Student Union.

The Jewish Student Union was housed in a building that had belonged to the Heidelberg Jewish community before the war. It was in a nice neighborhood with a garden, a kitchen, and a dining room.

"*We have at present 29 members — 8 girls and 21 boys,*" I wrote (in English) on behalf of the Jewish Student Union in an undated letter to a Jewish student organization at that time. "*Most of our members study medicine, some of them philosophy, dental medicine, chemistry and philology. A great deal of the students need only one or two more terms for their final examination.*"

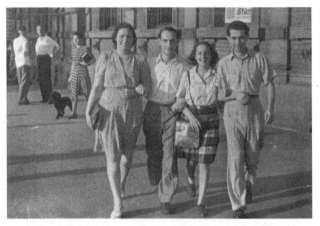

(From left) Lusia Hornstein, Max Zajac, Anna and Paul in
Heidelberg

Our number kept changing as some graduated or
emigrated and new refugees came — Jews from Poland,
Hungary, Czechoslovakia, and Germany who had survived
the war in hiding, or in forced labor battalions or in
concentration camps. We had all lost most of our families.
We were all in our twenties, eager to learn, and focused on
the future. Marcel introduced us to his soon-to-be-wife
Shoshana; to Max and Katie Zajac; to the Monias family
— a Jewish mother, father, son, and daughter — a rare
sight in those days. And we met Bob Lewis, an Army
dentist. He was married to Jo, who was born in Berlin,
deported to Auschwitz, and liberated in Bergen-Belsen.
She was adopted in the United States by the late Rabbi
Joachim Prinz. Bob had a big American car. The Lewises
took us and Steve and Lusia to many beautiful places in
Germany including Berchtesgaden.

There were also a few Americans who were medical students or with the Army who socialized with us. On Jewish holidays and Friday nights, we went to *Shabbat* services in a former German fraternity house that was now run by the American Army as a kind of community center for soldiers. Everyone spoke English there. I was introduced to Coca-Cola (which I loved), and both the Tuchmans and the Hornsteins got married on the premises. We had married in Hungary two years before, when no one we knew had a camera. Now, we, too, had a wedding portrait made.

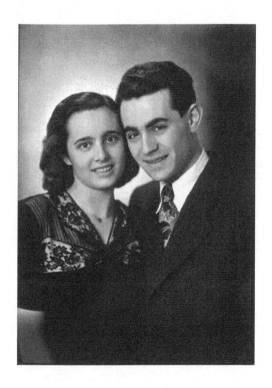

The friendships we developed at the Jewish Student Union in Heidelberg, even with those who ended up on different continents, were wonderful and have lasted our whole lives long. Almost everyone else, considered us a "problem."

As I wrote in my letter to a Jewish organization, we heard that in Palestine, there was an excess of "intelligentsia" and the countries willing to accept immigrants did not want foreign professionals but cheap laborers.

"We have tried from the first day after the liberation to get out of Germany as soon as possible and to resume our studies in the land of our destination. But in spite of our straining every nerve, only a very small fraction of our friends succeeded in doing so. We should like to stress the fact that although scores of German students went and are still going to Great Britain, Switzerland, Sweden, France, and even the United States, our chances have not increased.

"We take the liberty to put one question to you, reader: did you ever think about the above-mentioned problems and if so, what is your opinion?"

Paul H. Ornstein

*

In Heidelberg, I was finally able to reconnect to psychoanalysis and psychosomatic medicine. I was also in a seminar on psychotherapy, conducted by Professor Carl F.

Wendt — whose book on brief psychotherapy quoted all the "American" authors, especially Franz Alexander, who founded the Chicago Psychoanalytic Institute, where I would study after I emigrated to the U.S.

In Wendt's seminar I volunteered to present a discussion on one of Freud's papers. I approached Professor Wendt with the idea of doing my obligatory thesis *(Doctorarbeit)* with him on a psychotherapy-related topic but he advised me against it, saying I should work on something that could be completed sooner, to permit me to get to where I want to settle permanently.

He made the right suggestion.

I had another memorable experience at one of Professor Wendt's lectures. He brought in a young person, possibly 18 years old and interviewed him in front of us, asking us after the patient left the auditorium to discuss the clinical diagnosis. The class members suggested that the patient suffered from a severe compulsive neurosis. The patient was asked to return to the auditorium and was again interviewed.

After this interview the class suggested, without anyone dissenting, that the young man was suffering from paranoid schizophrenia. The point Professor Wendt wanted to bring home to us was that *the way we interview people matters as to what we get to see.* This is a lesson, the far-reaching impact of which it took me years to fully appreciate, when Heinz Kohut's ideas came on the scene.

*

After I finished medical school in 1950, I remained in

"Psychiatrische Klinik" for another year and did my dissertation on the use of nitrous oxide inhalation for the treatment of depression. I quickly obtained my medical doctors' degree and was prepared to leave Germany for the U.S.

Another outstanding experience belongs here, as it played a part in my development as a psychotherapist.

A young German assistant professor at the psychiatric clinic, Dr. Erich Hodel, became my good friend. There were some opportunities for such a friendship if a German colleague acknowledged that he knew what had happened to the Jews of Europe, rather than denying any knowledge. In this case, a trusting relationship could develop. Erich Hodel and I traveled to the Bodensee together for the "Lindauer Psychotherapie Woche" (the annual one-week meeting in Lindau) in 1950. We even shared a room, in order to be able to afford it.

There we were exposed to well-known psychotherapists, and witnessed an analytic-therapeutic session with a patient in front of a large audience. This left an unforgettable impression on me. It would give me the courage in my teaching of psychiatry residents to demonstrate analytically based psychotherapeutic interviews with patients and also to have them video-taped.

I should not underestimate the many ways in which living in the U.S. zone of Germany, rather than in communist Hungary between 1946 and 1951 affected our outlook on the world. We had access to news and information from every corner of the world, uncensored by communist propaganda and Stalinist distortions. We were avid readers of "*Die Zeit*" throughout our stay in Germany and read it even now when we visit Germany or any part

Europe. But, as much as we enjoyed our student years in Heidelberg, we were finally able to get refugee visas and, in June 1951, leave for the United States.

FIVE ~ United States

On June 28, 1951 we were on deck with countless others when we suddenly caught a glimpse of the Statue of Liberty. Our navy ship, the S.S. *General Ballou*, then transporting refugees from DP camps dropped anchor for the night just a short distance away. We could barely wait to disembark the next morning. I remember seeing the Statue of Liberty (which I had known only from picture postcards) for the first time, standing on deck transfixed, the image of Lady Liberty beginning to blur as tears of joy welled up in our eyes. We felt an intense gratitude for having been able to come to a country of incomparable freedom and opportunity. We felt truly liberated.

Of course, we felt liberated from the camps at the end of the war. We felt liberated when we crossed the border from Hungary to Austria; from there to the U.S. zone of Germany, liberated in stages, as if we could experience the intense excitement of regaining our lives only in small increments. Only one other time did Anna and I have a similarly intense experience to which our whole psychophysical organism reacted profoundly: that was our first arrival on a visit to Israel in 1959, to see my father and the country. Catching the view of Israel's coastline from the plane just before landing, the feeling of "homecoming" — even if only for a visit — put us in touch with *being a link in the chain in countless generations of Jews* and finally entering the country of our own. This was our "ultimate" liberation. Our joy was greatly enhanced by the fact that we brought our first child, six-year old daughter Sharone Beth, to visit her grandfather.

In New York in 1951, our reception by Anna's and my relatives made us feel immediately welcome. But it took a while to get settled in the new country, find work, and a place to pursue our psychiatric and psychoanalytic education.

First, I got an internship at Delaware State Hospital in Wilmington through the intervention of a Jewish army chaplain we met in Heidelberg, while Anna, who did not yet have her medical degree, worked as a nurses' helper. In Delaware, although I was an intern in general medicine, I treated my first psychiatric patient. He was scheduled for a lobotomy and he was known to be a very difficult, easily enraged patient, prone to attack people. No staff member wanted to tell him about his impending surgery but someone was needed to sit down with him and explain it.

The director, who was from Germany, suggested I do it. Although I had not yet been trained in psychiatry, I instinctively knew how to talk to the patient and he liked to talk to me. I prepared him for his lobotomy, introducing it in the course of a conversation that was close to hypnosis. It was a case of persuasion: my telling him what he had to undergo in order to get what he needed.

Today, the medical profession has realized that lobotomy was a poorly understood procedure that destroyed people's lives; in 1951, lobotomies were still regularly performed on violent or difficult patients in most mental hospitals in the U.S. and Europe. In my own training at the state mental hospitals where I interned, I learned the use of electro-shock treatments for mania, catatonia, or severe depression. Milder convulsions were induced by the use of insulin. The subject of my doctoral thesis had been the experimental use of nitrous oxide, a substance that also induced minor convulsions in patients with mild depression.

The first psychotropic medication, Thorazine, was introduced during my training in the early 1950s. The next few decades witnessed the rapid "medicalization" of psychiatry, which was difficult for me to accept. Psychoanalysts lost teaching positions in departments of psychiatry everywhere. I would publish several papers with my colleagues a decade later about the dangers of abandoning psychotherapy for the exclusive use of medication. Because of my commitment to psychoanalysis, I would never become proficient in the use of medications. But that is jumping ahead.

In January of 1952, I became an intern at Metropolitan Hospital on Welfare Island in New York City, while Anna went back to Heidelberg with Lusia Hornstein to finish medical school. (They had not graduated at the time we received our emigration visas to the United States). By the summer of 1952, we were reunited: Steve and I were residents, and Anna and Lusia, interns at Beth Israel Hospital in Newark, New Jersey.

As two refugee couples and four Jewish physicians who had survived the Nazis, we were written up in the *New York Times*.

It was in Newark, as a resident in internal medicine, that I experimented with hypnosis a little bit. I sometimes hypnotized guests at parties and nurses in their lounge —

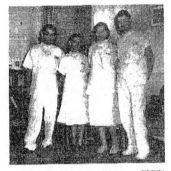

2 Refugee Couples, All Doctors,
Serve at Same Jersey Hospital

All on Staff of Beth Israel in Newark, They
Were Graduated From Heidelberg After
Getting Out of Nazi Death Camps

The New York Times, July 5, 1952

never alone because that would not have been appropriate! I would ask the person to lie down, close their eyes, and had some success.

So at Beth Israel, I was called in by a physician who knew of my interest and wanted me to try it out on his patient.

The patient was a very competent professional woman who worked as campaign manager for New Jersey Congressman Peter Rodino, later to become an important figure in the congressional hearings that led to the impeachment of President Richard Nixon. Rodino himself showed up at the hospital to talk to her doctor. He was running for re-election that November — less than three months off — and his campaign manager had suddenly been taken to Beth Israel, her legs apparently paralyzed, unable to walk.

The physician in charge of her could find nothing physically wrong. He was an internist with whom I did rounds once a week. He was aware of my interest in psychiatry and my particular interest in hypnosis. He asked me to take Rodino and his campaign manager off his hands. "Do what you need to do," he said.

I was pleased to be called in. I had been reading about the techniques of hypnosis since rabbinical school. By that fall of 1952, I was no longer an intern but a resident, and I thought I knew how to deal with patients.

The Congressman's campaign manager was in bed in her hospital room when I arrived. I asked her why she was there and how she felt and then, with her permission, I hypnotized her and was able to get her to tell me her story. As I understood it, she had been talking to a man on the telephone who was flirtatious with her and had tried to

87

seduce her. This attempt at seduction upset her so much that she couldn't move. I didn't have to be very knowledgeable to understand that she was suffering from a conversion disorder, in which psychological issues show themselves in physical form. I had read about this phenomenon back when I was a student at the Rabbinical Seminary with Zvi. And I understood you need to have an attitude and ability to deal with people so that they feel cared about and believe you can help them.

I met with her several times and with her boss, Congressman Rodino. After a few sessions, she was able to stand up and walk out of the hospital unassisted. He wanted her back on the campaign trail as soon as possible and came to thank me. What I had done was so important to him, he said, that if I ever needed something important, I should not hesitate to call. So I explained to him that I needed something right away: my mother-in-law was in Heidelberg waiting to immigrate and the list was very long. Rodino promised to speed matters up and he did.

Sophie arrived in the United States in November of the next year. The campaign manager herself was so grateful that she also wanted to return the favor and decided to teach me to drive. She brought her car to the hospital grounds, picked me up, sat next to me, and taught me how to drive her car. So I had my first driving lessons in New Jersey, and practiced more with colleagues during my residency in Waltham, Massachusetts, where I finally got my driver's license two years later.

Our time at Beth Israel was so important to us that we named our first daughter, Sharone Beth, after the hospital. She was born in May of 1953 and we were, of course, very happy to be new parents.

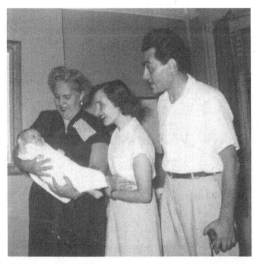

Rodino's campaign manager holding Sharone Beth

Anna had about six weeks left to finish her internship and since we lived at the hospital, we often left the baby in our room with instructions to all that if anyone heard her cry they should page Anna. Much of the hospital staff was involved with her care until we moved to Brooklyn, where I began a residency at Kings County Hospital.

Anna stayed home with Sharone until November when her mother Sophie arrived in the United States and took over Sharone's care so that Anna could go back to work. This was our most difficult time financially. I was studying with Steve for the New York State boards, but it turned out that the chairman had to be bribed in order for us to take them. It took me two meetings with him to figure this out and twelve more years before he was finally apprehended.

Very early on, we knew that it was very hard for

foreigners to be certified as physicians elsewhere in the United States. I had written postcards to every one of the 48 states asking if we could take the medical licensing exam there. I received replies from only five: New York, Ohio, Rhode Island, Illinois, and one other. Massachusetts was one of the states that was restrictive at the time. Nonetheless, in the summer of 1954, we moved to another Metropolitan Hospital in Waltham, Massachusetts.

We loved Boston and would have liked to remain there, but we could not qualify for the medical board and also I had a miserable experience at Harvard Medical School with Dr. Alvin Semrad.

I had the impression that, at Harvard, they were used to getting whatever and whomever they wanted. I had watched Semrad interview patients at Metropolitan hospital and thought he was very good at it. But when it came to interviewing me, he was totally silent. He said not one word, although he knew quite well why I was there. Finally, I told him I was leaving since he had nothing to say. I assume it was Semrad's way of indicating his lack of interest in me. Years later, we sat in the same row at an analytic meeting and he was very friendly. He no longer regarded me as a *shlemiel*.

After that experience in 1954, friends told me that I should try to get a psychiatric residency in Cincinnati. Ohio was one of the few states where I could take the medical exams and the Cincinnati training was known nationwide for its emphasis on long term psychoanalytically oriented psychotherapy. It was headed by Maurice Levine, a psychoanalyst himself, and one of the nation's noted psychiatric educators at that time. Cincinnati didn't take many foreigners but the way to do it, they said, was to try to meet with Dr. Levine. He would be attending the annual meeting of the American Psychiatric Association in Atlantic City.

I went to Atlantic City (to what was my first meeting of the APA) and met with him. Maurice Levine was about 50 and a very friendly person who told me he could not make such a decision himself. He invited me to come to Cincinnati for a visit, meet the group there, and then see.

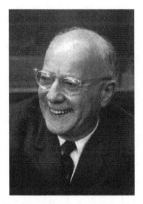

Dr. Maurice "Maury" Levine

My meetings went well and, four years after our arrival in the U.S., in June of 1955, Anna and I drove to Cincinnati to begin our residencies on July 1. Since we didn't know where we would live and had no furniture, Sophie flew with Sharone to Chicago, where Steve was working for a GP and Lusia was taking care of her own baby, while we got settled.

This was a forward-looking time for America with Dwight D. Eisenhower in the White House. I felt very much a part of the optimistic, positive spirit of the country. Also, at the time of our arrival, psychodynamic psychiatry and psychoanalysis were at their zenith. American culture supported the psychoanalytic ethos: it was portrayed in literature, movies, and theater. Thousands of Americans were being analyzed or had been analyzed.

We had arrived in the U.S. at the right time.

SIX ~ Cincinnati

For our first two years in Cincinnati, we lived in an apartment with minimal furnishings. There, Anna and I studied for the licensing boards. Anna read the material out loud and I often fell asleep while she was reading, but I had the idea that I could absorb the material anyway. When I took the Ohio boards, I placed first in the state.

Then we began to look for a house. We found a large, well-built, old house in a beautiful neighborhood not far from the hospital and downtown Cincinnati. The seller was a woman who had grown up in the house and had inherited it from her parents. Her husband did not want her to sell it. They were asking $42,000 — too much for me.

So I waited. I thought: it was *her* house; it should be her decision. The fact that she hated what she had inherited made it easy for me to bargain.

In the end, I got it at a good price — approximately $28,000 and took out a mortgage. In November of 1959, we moved to 4177 Rose Hill Avenue.

Our first and only house in America was beautiful, and more than large enough to accommodate our growing family.

Our daughter Miriam Lilla was born in 1958, when we still lived in an apartment. Rafael David was born in 1960.

Until she died a year later of cancer, Anna's mother, Sophie, helped us by cooking and caring for the children.

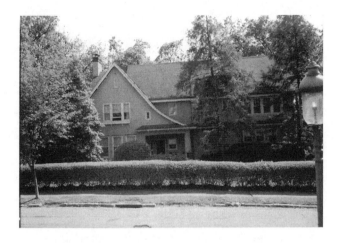

My father had remarried, learned Hebrew, found work and was living happily in Israel, just north of Haifa. Margit came from a Hajdúnánás family; my father had known her and her four children before the war. Her Zionist husband had died in a labor battalion during the war.

After my father arrived in Israel, he visited them so frequently that her oldest daughter finally suggested that they get married. I didn't particularly like Margit — I thought she was not an equal intellectual partner for him — but it was better for my father to be married than to live alone.

He realized, as we did, that conditions in Israel at the time could not offer Anna and me the opportunities we had in the United States.

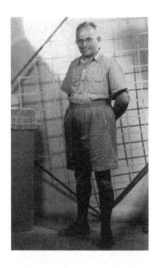

Our positions at the University of Cincinnati were secure; our academic advancement seemed to be a certainty; it looked like both of us would be promoted from instructors to assistant and associate to full professors. Another major move just seemed impossible to undertake and that created a deep inner struggle for me. Anna and I felt it was a betrayal of the Zionist cause, a betrayal of our life-long ideals, a betrayal of what we would now call our "nuclear self." Zionism was certainly one of the building blocks of my nuclear self and not having moved to Israel is something I shall never be able to live down.

My father's acceptance of our decision to remain in Cincinnati was very helpful to me. He had always tried to understand my interests and wishes. Long before I became a psychoanalyst, I had told him a great deal about my interest in psychoanalysis. In Israel, my father met Zvi and his brother — the rabbinical school students who first got me interested in it. We would make many family visits to my father in Israel; he and Margit would come to Cincinnati; we would frequently meet in Europe and travel to places in Italy and Switzerland we had only dreamt about before. These trips were educational and very exciting for our children. I still remember Rafael's unhappiness when I told him we didn't have time to see the Forum Romanum. But he insisted and we did.

We and the Hornsteins all wanted to live in the same place, so all our children could grow up together, as Steve and I had done in Hajdúnánás. In 1956, the Hornsteins were living in Chicago. Steve had applied for an interview for an Ob/GYN residency in Cincinnati but gynecology at the University of Cincinnati was part of the Department of Surgery and, before 1956, it had never accepted a Jew for training. He was told that all residents' positions had already been filled for the year.

Luckily, the Dean of our Medical School was aware that I had placed first on the Ohio State Medical Boards. He had congratulated me in person, and, like Congressman Rodino said if there was ever anything he could help me with, to call him up. At that point, I told him that I had a good friend with whom I had gone to medical school who was brilliant but unable to get an interview at our university because of some old-fashioned attitudes. The Dean looked into the matter, Steve was then able to obtain an interview, did very well, and was offered an appointment as an Ob/GYN resident starting in the summer of 1956. Lusia became a resident in Pediatrics at Cincinnati's Children's Hospital. They moved into a house just one house away from ours.

Every Passover, our two families held a joint Seder, which Steve and I conducted together the way we remembered our fathers had done.

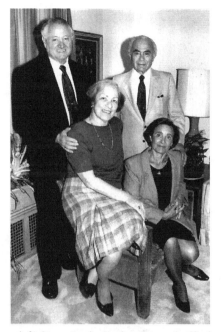

(From left) Steve, Lusia, Paul and Anna in Cincinnati

Although I didn't go through all the rooms of our house with a feather looking for *chametz* as he had done in Hungary, I tried to conduct the Seder as my father had done. That's what I learned to do and I continued with it. In addition to all the Jewish holidays, we celebrated Thanksgiving, and all our birthdays with the Hornsteins.

As I look back on it, settling in Cincinnati was in many ways a felicitous choice. From the beginning, we were very happy there. It was then a prosperous Midwestern city of about half a million people. We lived in a largely Jewish neighborhood. We became naturalized American citizens in 1956, made good friends, liked to go shopping downtown, to restaurants and to the theater. By the late 1950s, we both spoke fairly good English. I read the newspapers every day: *The New York Times* and the *Cincinnati Enquirer*. When we arrived in New York, Anna and I had decided: "From here on, we speak only English." We tried never to speak a word of Hungarian to our children and tried to speak as little Hungarian as possible with Sophie. We all believed that we needed to learn English as well and as quickly as we had learned German.

The department of psychiatry in which I trained for three years and in which I ascended the academic ladder from instructor in 1957 to full professor in 1970 was a psychoanalytically-oriented training center within the Cincinnati General Hospital — the University of Cincinnati's main teaching hospital. The Chairman, Professor Maurice Levine, was himself a psychoanalyst. We were encouraged to take on two or three patients for long-term psychotherapy under supervision, and work with them for the entire three years of training — an impossibility later in the age of "managed care." Anna became part of the department of Child Psychiatry and became a full Professor in 1976.

The medical school included a community clinic where anyone could walk in and receive treatment. I saw patients who were black and white, young and old, rich and poor, some for just a session or two, some for a long time. Since we psychiatric residents weren't paid much, we were also allowed to see private patients at the hospital and charge them privately. Soon I settled into a regular schedule. From eight until noon every weekday, I saw patients. Then again from two to six. On Thursdays, we residents had a weekly lunch seminar. On the other days, five or six of us residents had lunch together, discussing the events of the day as well as issues that had come up with patients. It was a very friendly group.

Maurice Levine lived up to his reputation. He created a very friendly atmosphere in the department, organizing parties in his home and picnics in nearby parks. He was Jewish, a native of Cincinnati, and one of the first psychoanalytically trained psychiatrists in the country to be appointed a department chairman. His book, *Psychotherapy in Medical Practice (1942)*, was translated into many languages and he wrote a special chapter on psychotherapy in Franz Alexander's *Dynamic Psychiatry,* subdividing treatment into supportive-, suppressive-, relationship-, and exploratory- or insight-psychotherapy. This division is no longer tenable today but Levine's description of each form, the details of how each was to be conducted, stood the test of time — if we look at the *process* of therapy, in which each of these supposedly discrete approaches do have their place. Levine emphasized relationship-psychotherapy: his goal was that after completing training, we should all be able to sustain a long-term, therapeutic relationship with patients and he also encouraged us to seek psychoanalytic training.

In spite of his adherence to Freudian drive theory in his psychoanalytic practice, he had an idea about the human psyche unusual in the profession then: that every human being is born with a "basic goodness" at the core of his or her being. Surrounding this core, Levine believed, was a layer of anxiety, born of conflict, leading to the next layer, the layer of defenses which manifested itself in the patient's often obnoxious, problematic behavior. He advised us to look beneath the defensive layer to the underlying conflict and anxiety. Well anchored theoretically, or not, it created a culture of respect for the patient that was emblematic of the Cincinnati training. This idea of basic goodness, incidentally, had already been important in Ferenczi's psychoanalytic theories, then in Balint's, and even more profoundly in Kohut's self psychology.

Aside from trainees doing psychotherapy under supervision by staff-psychiatrists, Levine provided an intellectual atmosphere in the department by frequently inviting guest lecturers and visiting professors, who would spend some time each year in residence. Among these were the anthropologist Margaret Mead, the philosopher Abraham Kaplan, the psycho-pharmacologist-existential therapist Heinz Lehmann, the psychoanalysts Phillip Seitz and Joseph Kepecs.

I always volunteered to be the one to pick up our visitors at the airport. It was about an hour away and it gave me a chance to be with them alone. At the time, there was no security and the custom was to walk onto the tarmac and wait as the passengers got out of the airplane. One of the first visitors was Margaret Mead. I didn't know how to greet her so when a large, elegantly-dressed woman came towards me, I instinctively kissed her hand.

"Hungarian!" she diagnosed me immediately.

Knowing that she was a famous anthropologist, I had worried about what we would talk about on the way back. She had been a good friend of the Levines and I knew she was a very important anthropologist. But there was no problem: she was a person who liked to talk to you more than she liked to listen. She used to come to Cincinnati for several years, for two weeks each time. We became good friends and she would have dinner at our home on all her visits. The children would invite their friends to come.

They sat on the living room floor while she talked to them, always while she was knitting. Margaret loved a good argument and discussions with her were always very instructive, especially about current events. I remember arguing with her about the existence of the State of Israel. That issue remained and still remains important to me.

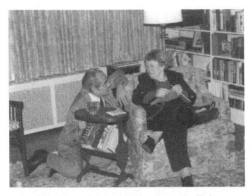

Paul with Margaret Mead in the Ornstein living room

In order to further enrich our experiences, once a month, throughout the academic year, one of the professors of English Literature at the university would discuss a novel or a play that would be performed in Cincinnati. One of these professors was James Robinson who had been a student of the poet Robert Frost. Or, a psychiatrist or psychoanalyst on the faculty like Stanley Kaplan, would create psychoanalytic profiles of characters of a selected play that was being performed in one of the local theaters. Once a week, throughout the academic year, the noon hour on Thursdays was devoted to presentations by guests from other departments of the university (sociology, history, philosophy, law and others). The emeritus professor of physiology and noted writer Gustav Eckstein was a steady "fixture" at Grand Rounds and other teaching sessions. All of these opportunities for learning created a stimulating atmosphere in the department — a distinctive advantage for someone embarking on a psychiatric-psychoanalytic career. I participated enthusiastically in these endeavors and repeatedly tried out my developing ideas in these contexts.

*

When I was a second-year trainee in 1956, Michael and Enid Balint began their regular visits to Cincinnati at Levine's initiative. The very first visit was a revelation to Anna and me. We suddenly realized what psychoanalytic psychotherapy could be like, even before we began our psychoanalytic training.

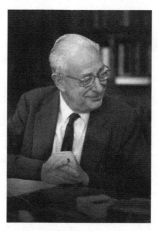

Michael Balint

Balint was very well known at the time. Naturally, I volunteered to pick him up at the airport. He had lived in England after getting out of Hungary in time. Michael Balint was born Bergsmann in Budapest in 1896 and converted from Judaism to Unitarian Christianity. He was 60 then and I was 32 when we met. I spoke a little Hungarian with him. We had much in common, and he liked my entire family. I didn't like the way he had changed his name and left his Jewishness behind, but I was deeply influenced by several aspects of the way he practiced psychotherapy.

Balint never called his brand of psychoanalytic theory (which was object relations theory) anything but plain psychoanalysis. He seemed to me more "human," less rigid, and less rule-bound and formulaic than was usual then. In the clinical dialogue, Balint seemed guided by what the patient signaled he or she wanted or needed from him. What he demonstrated behind the one-way mirror when he was teaching us was his close attention to the dialogue between patient and therapist. His interpretations came across as natural conversation, whose plausibility we could easily grasp — even if we could not immediately emulate it.

Because Balint focused on how the patient related to him in session, he was unwilling to listen to any prolonged descriptions of our patient's history when we presented our cases in supervision or in clinical seminars. He wanted to hear the actual dialogue without much background. He was interested in *how* the past history became *interwoven in the dialogue*. Balint did not want to interpret the *history as such,* or assess the patient's problems on the basis of the history. Instead, he focused his attention on the patient's current experience with the therapist that would disclose what ailed him or her *now*. The meaning of the history seemed to emerge more naturally in the context of the dialogue and his interpretations appeared less imposed on the clinical data. Our experiences in doing psychotherapy henceforth became more alive, more affect-laden and more affect-mobilizing. My exposure to the Balints' approach during their annual visits was a transformative experience in the process of my development as a psychotherapist.

Balint's idea of a "basic fault" which he proposed in his book *The Basic Fault* (1962) had a lasting impact on Anna's and my own psychoanalytic development. By conceptualizing the basic fault as occurring in early infantile and childhood development, Balint opened up for us pre-oedipal problems for *psychoanalytic* scrutiny. He did not supply us with equally penetrating, explicit treatment principles, but described the necessary clinical atmosphere that had to prevail in the treatment setting. Balint's *descriptions* of the transferences established by patients with a basic fault are unsurpassed to this day and his work in this area prepared us for Heinz Kohut's comprehensive and theoretically more compelling contributions as well as treatment principles. Balint insisted that the issue in the basic fault was not *conflict* but *a fault*, which resulted from the unavailability of the necessary caretaker responsiveness.

The Balints came to Cincinnati almost every year from 1956 through 1970. They wanted to move from England permanently and to work in our department and Maurice Levine was at first quite excited about this idea, but there were problems. Levine, in his old-fashioned way, thought that social workers like Enid Balint should only work with other social workers, and he excluded her from our seminars. Enid wanted to be acknowledged as a psychoanalyst. I viewed her that way. I liked and respected both Balints and sometimes even preferred Enid's ideas. Sometimes the two of us even ganged up on her husband! I was sorry not to have them in Cincinnati, but they remained very important to Anna and me, and we visited them in London, and had a few days of vacation with them in Italy.

In one of his early visits, Michael Balint and I discussed his work with psychiatrists on focal psychotherapy. He showed me that *brevity* did not need to be at the expense of *depth* when the principles of psychoanalysis were adapted to the shorter time frame and the focus for interpretive comments were formulated early in the treatment. In the course of these conversations, Balint asked me to join him in writing a book about focal psychotherapy. I spent six weeks working with him and his wife on the book in the Dolomite Mountains. For me, this was a most memorable experience.

After he died suddenly in 1971, I received a letter from London inviting me to write a paper for a *Festschrift* for him. I decided that the most appropriate paper would be to write up a patient I had treated with his method. The "fireman," as we referred to this working class man in his 30s, with a wife and five children, was assigned to me as a patient. He was in deep pain because his wife had had an affair. When he discovered it, rather impulsively he decided to divorce her, and developed a serious depression with an inability to eat or sleep. The clinic provided only six sessions of psychotherapy with a follow-up and I thought that he was a good candidate on whom to test Balint's principles of focal therapy.

When I contacted him six months later for his follow-up, I could hear him excitedly telling his wife, "It's my doctor! It's my doctor!"

He told me that the brief period of psychotherapy had helped him become a better husband and father. He had decided to remain in his marriage and he felt better able to communicate with his wife about what he wanted and needed.

This paper for Balint's *Festschrift* marked the beginning of Anna's and my long professional collaboration. I had audio-taped the six-session treatment and the six-month follow-up with the patient's consent. Now I asked Anna to listen to the tapes and determine what led to the striking clinical improvement. She would be able to look at the course of this focal therapy with another pair of eyes and determine if I had followed Balint's principles correctly. It was an important project for us. We discovered that we could draw on one another's ideas and capacities in the writing. The paper "Focal Psychotherapy: Its potential Impact on Psychotherapeutic Practice in Medicine" was published in *Psychiatry in Medicine* in 1972: our first joint paper.

Balint's most significant influence on me, however, were our many discussions about *The Basic Fault.* Much later, in 1992, I was asked by the publisher to write a preface to a new edition of his book.

The concept of the basic fault refers to a discrepancy in the formative years between the infant's basic needs and the response of the caregivers. This creates a state of deficiency in the structure of the developing psyche.

Balint replaced Freud's idea of *primary narcissism,* which assumes that others don't exist for the infant at the beginning of extra-uterine life, with *primary love,* which assumes that from the very beginning of life there is a primary form of relatedness to others. He said that a common feature of all these primitive forms of object relationship is that the object is taken for granted — only one partner may have wishes, interests, demands on the other. This primary relatedness is the cornerstone of Balint's ideas, with many implications. Sadism, hate and the manifestations of narcissism are always to be considered as secondary.

Like Kohut would later do, Balint used his patient's language and imagery to describe the nature of the basic fault — which is felt as a fault, not a complex or conflict or situation. Its cause is a previous failure on the part of another person and therefore the patient is expressing a desperate demand that this time the analyst should not fail him. The treatment situation must allow for a regression to the level of the basic fault. The analyst then "has to be with the patient" to allow for a new beginning. The central ideas in *The Basic Fault* are congruent with the self psychology I would learn about from Kohut. So Balint's book prepared me for Kohut's *The Analysis of the Self.*

*

Given the richness of my professional life, my satisfaction with Cincinnati and my overall psychiatric training as well as with my steady advancement on the academic ladder, it is hard to explain why I also felt a growing dissatisfaction.

The psychotherapy we were taught, mainly in supervision and clinical conferences — there were no formal lectures on theory and practice — emphasized a watered-down notion of the therapeutic relationship as the matrix of the curative process. You talked about your therapeutic relationship with your supervisor. Every quarter, your supervisor changed and was not always a faculty member, but sometimes a psychiatrist from another hospital in the city or a psychiatrist from the community. Nobody was terrible but some were sort of flat, and one was strange. I had to sit a certain physical distance away from him when we met for supervision. I expected all of them to be insightful and to be able to draw me out about my interactions with my patients. None of my supervisors in Cincinnati were able to do that well.

The psychotherapy we were taught put less emphasis on a systematic interpretation of preconscious derivatives of unconscious content than on the relationship. This was guided by a somewhat superficial ego psychological narrative of elements of the oedipal relations to authority figures. It seemed to me that a "formula" guided our dialogue with patients. I felt that I had brought with me to the therapeutic task a pre-existing capacity to establish and maintain a long-term "relationship" — I was looking for something more specific, to guide me in conducting a more meaningful psychotherapeutic dialogue with my patients. Psychoanalytically *oriented* psychotherapy (in my book) was not yet *psychoanalytic* psychotherapy.

At first, Anna found it easier to be flexible than I did. Nobody among my psychotherapy patients ever called me at my home. Late one night, after we had gone to bed, a patient anxious about traveling to Florida called me at home and said he thought he was having a heart attack. Not fully awake, I said, "What do you want me to do?" Anna kicked me and said, "That's no way to talk to a patient!" So I asked him what he was worried about. He told me he wasn't sure he should go to Florida. We talked for a while and his anxiety decreased; and he made the trip.

The patient reported back to me later that my matter-of-fact tone of voice and my lack of concern regarding the possibility of his having a heart attack relieved his anxiety and he had been able to enjoy his vacation. I was pleased but very puzzled at that time in my training about our inability to know specifically how our patients were experiencing what we said and how we said it.

Many of the instructors and assistant professors in the department flew to Chicago every other weekend (during the academic year) for psychoanalytic training at the Chicago Psychoanalytic Institute, for coursework and supervision. They had their personal analyses in Cincinnati. There were four training analysts in our own Department of Psychiatry.

I also wanted to get my psychoanalytic training, of course, but at first I could afford neither the time nor the money for what was a five-year curriculum, with a comprehensive exam at the end of it. There were other hurdles as well. First, you had to be accepted. Candidates from Denver, Cincinnati and St. Louis (where there were no local institutes at the time) applied to Chicago. The entire process was somewhat mysterious. Several people I knew had applied to the Institute but were not accepted and never understood why.

It didn't occur to me that I would not be accepted. I had wanted to be a psychoanalyst already in Rabbinical Seminary and all through the war and in Germany. My working with the Balints had made me very comfortable with psychoanalytic techniques. I thought that I deserved to be accepted.

Six people interviewed me at a conference table, three on each side, myself at the head. These were my prospective teachers: two women and four men. Other people who had gone through this process told me that they would ask me what I was doing in Cincinnati and what my "issues," i.e. problems, were, but I didn't know what they wanted to hear, or what was acceptable or not acceptable to say. The interview lasted about an hour to ninety minutes.

I don't remember the details anymore but I know my examiners wanted to know something about my neurosis. I didn't think I had one, but in any case, we weren't expected to be able to spell it out ourselves. They went about it trying to elicit our family history.

I didn't tell them that I didn't think I needed a personal analysis. I said that I had wanted to become a psychoanalyst since I was very young and interested in the workings of the mind. I was applying for a personal analysis because it was required by the Institute. My examiners were a little bit side-tracked by the fact that I was a refugee of the Second World War, and they asked me questions about that.

I was not a typical war refugee, I told them. The war had affected me greatly because I lost my mother, my sister, my brothers, and other members of my family, but I had been in a labor battalion — not a concentration camp — and I had not felt personally degraded by the Nazis. Instead, I degraded them; I had a kind of bullet-proof vest to protect my self-esteem as a Jew. But I told my examiners that I had seen other people with other kinds of responses. I had seen Jews whose feelings of humiliation killed them. I was also lucky in that I was physically never in circumstances where I could have died.

This was not entirely true. I could have been killed on the front line during *katyusha* fire and many times on the streets of Budapest when I was out on the streets in defiance of the curfew.

Some people found this group interview traumatizing; I did not. They accepted me and in the fall of 1959, 20 years after I first became interested in psychoanalysis, I was finally able to begin my course of formal study.

SEVEN ~ Chicago

Chicago was 300 miles away from Cincinnati and, at that time, it took nearly a day to drive there. The only way to commute efficiently was to fly. It wasn't so expensive — the airplane ticket cost $11 — but it took time to drive to the airport, fly to Chicago, get to the hotel room which cost $9 — and while you gained an hour flying there, you lost an hour when you returned. Luckily, I was able to have my personal psychoanalysis in Cincinnati.

I was also fortunate in my analyst: Louis A. Gottschalk was an American who was both an adult and child psychoanalyst. A pioneering neuroscientist who had trained at the Chicago Institute for Psychoanalysis and subsequently moved to Cincinnati, he was a senior professor in the Department of Psychiatry and later became Founding Chairman of the Department of Psychiatry and Human Behavior at the University of California, Irvine Medical School. Then, I often thought that it might have been his child-analytic training that made him less dogmatic and rigid than other analysts I have known.

During my first session, he asked me to describe myself in writing and to leave it with him. I had never heard of that being done by anyone before but I did it. I no longer remember exactly what I wrote but I must have written about Judit's death, and about my mother and three younger brothers being deported to Auschwitz. Prior to the analysis, I was constantly thinking about them. I was always very much aware of what I lost. But I thought: life has to continue; I have to live. The details of my family in Hungary did not get center stage in my analysis.

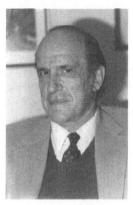

Dr. Louis A. Gottschalk

Actually, I didn't think I was sick enough for analysis! Of course, when you begin to learn about your inner world, it can bring new things to light, but I no longer remember what those things were. I only discussed my analysis with Anna and we were both so busy that neither of us went into much detail.

I thought Gottschalk resembled my father in his eloquence. He was widely read, with a broad perspective on life. He was good at interpreting dreams. He liked to link the dream to an earlier experience or theme rather than interpret the dream without its context. My analyst never seemed to repeat himself. What he said always seemed relevant to the moment. He listened to me and not to his theory (as I perceived it) and had one other remarkable characteristic: his interpretations were never assertions of a favored "hobby-horse." They were fresh and context-dependent; not generalized or routine, dynamic formulations — with few exceptions that I can recall.

Some of these exceptions are vivid in my mind because these were so unusual: on one occasion, at the end of his summer vacation, as Dr. Gottschalk arrived at his office for my first post-vacation session, I happened to be at the glass-door, where he entered. Seeing him coming I opened the door with obvious satisfaction at his return. At some point in the session that followed, he interpreted my eagerness to open the door for him so politely, as a way to deny my "rage" at him for having been away for the month of August.

I thought that was ridiculous for two reasons. First, he did not understand the culturally ingrained behavior of my upbringing in Hungary: every Hungarian boy is raised to hold the door for older people. Second, I felt truly pleased to see him again after my own pleasant vacation with my family. He listened to my objections and while he didn't seem to accept my cultural explanation, he didn't argue. The theory of "reaction formation" (turning a feeling into its opposite) got the better of him, but at least he did not "push" his interpretation at a time when others would have insisted that I was resisting their "correct" interpretations.

My four years on the couch (five times and later four times a week), did not give me much of a chance to *observe* "the analytic *process.*" I was too involved in it for that. Calling it a *training analysis* was a misnomer. It is true that from time to time, and certainly after I completed it and when I was beginning to do analysis myself, episodes of what I experienced and what my analyst did or said — his interpretations — occasionally came back to me before they faded away almost completely. I didn't retain it — it was gone. Only the results of the analysis remained with me. I understood what may have led to my teenage shyness; and to my anxiety in public speaking, in competitive poetry recitals (in gymnasium and in rabbinical school) — where I was always frightened that I would not recall my lines. I knew that my wish to shine and be admired in those activities had something to do with it — these were not unconscious, their deeper roots may well have been — along with the fact that I could not picture reaching the level of my father's oratory which I greatly admired and wished to emulate.

I liked my analyst. I knew him quite well because he was my colleague, a member of the faculty at my hospital. Every year there was a Christmas party; every summer an outing to the country with a picnic; so I could interact with him in an informal setting as well as at work. I thought Dr. Gottschalk was a good man, but I didn't put him up on a pedestal in the way I idealized Balint and, later, Kohut. And there was another thing: some analysands have no one they can talk to the way they can talk to their analyst. I could talk in this way to my wife.

The termination of my analysis was not traumatic either. There should be a pleasurable feeling of finishing an experience but it inevitably echoes other terminations. I was lucky in this too. I set the date after four years for some five months ahead. Some new insights emerged, but I felt I could explore them on my own and that Gottschalk didn't have much new to say. I may have told him, "I think I'm pretty much done. So maybe we stop just before you go on summer vacation?" That's what we did.

I felt freed up and relieved that it was over. I could now

devote my energy to my patients and my work although I knew that inner work is never over.

There is no such thing as a complete analysis. "Complete" means that you are able to continue the habit of reflectiveness that you have developed with the analyst. If you work as a psychoanalyst, you never stop finding out more about yourself because each new patient draws in a different aspect of you in order to be in touch with them.

My self-reflection was triggered again and again with each new patient I worked with. I learned something from all of them. But when I began training as a psychoanalyst, I worried that my patients wouldn't find the psychoanalytic process as painless as I did. I also worried that given my war experience, I wouldn't be empathic enough to small neurotic complaints — I would not be able to appreciate personal trauma because of my experience undergoing apocalyptical trauma: losing my mother, my sister and my three brothers. But I found out very soon that any kind of trauma could affect someone in a profound way.

*

I began flying to classes at the Chicago Institute for Psychoanalysis every other week in the fall of 1960. I drove myself to the airport on Thursday evenings after work, or sometimes very early Friday morning. Classes ran from Friday morning until evening. Then the ten or so of us candidates went out to dinner together and then to sleep. On Saturday, there were more classes from eight to noon, then a bus to the airport and then back to Cincinnati.

The Institute was located on Michigan Avenue in

downtown Chicago. It was founded by Franz Alexander, a Hungarian Jew born in Budapest in 1891. He had studied with Karen Horney and Helene Deutsch at the Berlin Psychoanalytic Institute under Karl Abraham. In 1930, the President of the University of Chicago invited Alexander to teach there and he helped establish the second oldest (after New York) analytic institute in the U.S. By the time I arrived, Alexander had left Chicago for California and I met him only once.

Levine had invited him to be part of the series of famous people who came to speak to us and, as I was the designated driver to the airport, I was invited to breakfast with Alexander at a very fancy hotel downtown where such important visitors were lodged. I had never eaten at the restaurant at that hotel but, as it happened, one of my former patients was a waiter there. He had come to the clinic with an alcohol problem, had overcome it, and been able to take this relatively good job. He called me "Dr. Ornstein" and talked to me more than was usual. Alexander noticed and asked me if I ate there frequently. I did not divulge the truth of how the waiter and I knew one another.

I had the required four supervised cases: 200 hours were the minimum for completion. I wrote about them in "Selected Problems in Learning How to Analyze" published in *The International Journal of Psychoanalysis* in 1967. That paper is a window onto how I was thinking at the time. I began it by noting that psychoanalytic training evolved from an initially rather informal preceptorship to a complex tripartite system of personal analysis; courses in theory and technique; and supervised analysis. Formal supervision was introduced in 1920 at the Berlin Institute.

An inevitable problem in learning how to analyze, I wrote, stems from the fact that initially the student analyst has only a vague notion about what the analytic process is. His or her own analysis is usually still in progress and his coursework gives him only a fragmented view of the process. So much emphasis is placed on how the patient on the couch feels, that it is easy to lose sight of the student sitting behind him or her. How does the analyst feel? I asked.

"Sitting behind the patient may have been a comfortable solution for Freud," I wrote back then, "but it is not immediately comfortable for the beginner, whose successful transactions with others have up to now occurred face to face. Freud wanted to avoid being looked at, but the supervisee cannot do so; he is constantly being watched by his supervisor. Not having full grasp of the situation and the process, the recurrent, intrusive "What am I supposed to do?" leads to a considerable loss of spontaneity. Under such circumstances, while prepared for the role of relative passivity, such as non-manipulative, non-acting, non-advising, non-directing, etc., nevertheless, old non-analytic modes of response threaten to break through and often do...

"The difficulty in citing a distinct example of a learning problem and its successful resolution from this first phase stems from the fact that in my experience these problems were diffuse, their solution gradual, imperceptible, often occurring much later. Also, *how to feel as an analyst* is much harder to conceptualize and describe than how to behave, talk, think, and listen... This difficulty is by no means adequately described under the heading of counter-transference."

In addition to learning *how to feel as an analyst*, I needed to learn *how to behave and talk as an analyst*. "The beginner is even more self-conscious about the manner and content of his verbal communications than about his non-verbal behavior," I wrote. "He sees the former as a formidable task and soon becomes preoccupied with what is the correct phrasing, timing, brevity or length of his interpretations or confrontations. His special difficulty arises in connection with keeping content and process apart and wondering when to focus on one or the other, when not to interpret and what not to interpret."

A third part of my paper dealt with *how to think as an analyst*; a fourth with *how to listen with evenly suspended attention* — which can be as difficult for the analyst as free association is for the analysand. At first there seemed to be a bewildering number of frames of reference or areas to focus on in the analytic situation and process. Note taking, the need to have all the data for supervision and presentation at clinical conferences may interfere with analytic listening. But, more important, the student analyst fears that by not directing his attention to anything in particular, he will not find an anchor from which he can intervene interpretively.

Looking back from a distance of 50 years, I can say that I learned something about how to analyze from all four of my supervisors — not always what they wanted me to learn, and not from what they actually said, *but from my experiences with them*, whether positive or negative.

My first supervisor, Helen V. McLean, was a gracious lady who had a reputation for being erudite and was very good at listening. I felt that she was always with me, but contributed little explicitly to my learning how to analyze. What I finally understood was that she wanted me to express myself as fully as possible. This was very helpful to me and I also enjoyed it. Her attitude alone was encouraging to me. I always felt I would have liked to hear something specific from her about my conduct of my first analysis of a young, single nurse whom I called G.G.

She was a good first analysand: about 25 years old, cheerful, good-looking, who came into analysis because of depression following the break-up of her engagement and her recognition that she was unable to get along with men. I was looking forward to finally being able to actually do what I had been preparing to do for so long! I started by asking G.G. a few basic questions, then suggested that she lie down on the couch.

Helen McLean said very little to me during supervision. At the time, I did not appreciate her concept of supervision and I could not understand why she had almost nothing to add to what I had reported. Only later did I value the fact that she let me be and find my own way. She approved my starting with my second patient in a timely fashion.

My second analytic supervisor and my favorite was the Dean of the Education at the Institute, Joan Fleming. Many supervisees had difficult times with her. I, however, found her benign and very helpful. My second patient was a married man in his late thirties, the father of three children. Joan was good at drawing me out on the meaning of my experiences with my patient, the nature of his psychopathology and the details of my interventions. She also led me to higher levels of abstraction from my clinical data. One of her supervisory techniques was to draw me out to think more about what I have brought to our sessions. She injected her own ideas only when I reported something whose meaning I did not discern. Her method enlarged my own perspective about my patient. Because she followed the sequence of what I presented to her every other week — and she had a remarkable memory for the details — she taught me about the process of analysis by example. I learned that in analysis certain themes might seem to be random as part of free associations but there is always a connecting link, a continuity, to what the patient experiences on the emotional level of the communication.

My interest in the meaning of the *analytic process* itself began with Balint, was reinforced by my work with Fleming and then became a central concern of mine throughout my professional life. The patient whose analysis Fleming supervised terminated his analysis *"lege artis,"* (according to the rules, or properly) a short time before my first patient did.

Both women knew how to teach and let me be at the same time. They created a good climate for supervision. My two male supervisors did not.

My third supervisor was Samuel D. Lipton, a respected analyst, not a faculty member of the Institute but on the list of supervisors. He wanted primarily to teach me the way *he* was doing analysis, and was less interested or less accepting of how I was doing it — but we got along well because I wanted to learn from him. My patient was a married man with two children, an executive and a frustrated writer. He found it difficult to fit into a branch of the family business, where an older man was in charge. My patient had a variety of difficult problems that emerged in the context of a deepening process that I did not adequately understand.

Neither did my supervisor, although he thought he did. I could not really engage the patient on the basis of what my supervisor understood and suggested for me to do. At Lipton's suggestion, I told my patient that his choice of black prostitutes for his extramarital relations had to do with his need for these women to be so very different from his mother. He felt drawn to such women even though he was terrified that he might be discovered and disgraced because only with them could he have sexual pleasures. No matter how I phrased my understanding, he experienced my comments (and rightly so — as I later realized) as my opinion that he should stop seeing such women. Finally, unexpectedly, the patient quit his analysis. Neither I, nor my supervisor understood why. Only much later, in the course of the fifth, private supervision I sought out with Heinz Kohut did I belatedly understand what exactly happened. This was also true for my fourth supervised analysis.

My fourth supervisor was Hermann M. Serota, who also "knew" what I should learn from him. I was warned by other trainees not to undergo supervision from Serota because his response after only one or two sessions was: "You need more analysis!"

That warning was correct but my response was firm: "I just finished my analysis a few months ago. If I feel the need for it again, I will know what to do."

My fourth patient was a smart, competitive woman psychologist, referred to me by my former analyst Louis Gottschalk, married to a less accomplished man and dissatisfied. My supervisor interpreted her competitiveness as "penis-envy," about which he stated some generalities. That didn't sit right with me but I didn't know what to do about it. He kept urging me to have more analysis. I said, quite firmly, that the issue was not more analysis. I needed to learn something from him *in relation to my patient.* After that he stopped pestering me and we got along fairly well. This patient also left her analysis without my supervisor's or my own adequate, deeper understanding of the reasons for it.

I was able to learn something from both of my male supervisors though I sometimes found them impossible. They wanted me to accept what they taught without question. They had their own ideas of what I should focus on without hearing what I conveyed of what the patient told me. Since I had to complete four analyses to graduate, I tried my best to make sense of their supervision. But on Friday nights, when the candidates met for dinner and gossiped about their supervisors, I learned that these two were known to want to produce clones of themselves. I couldn't tell them that; I didn't argue with them. But the analyses I conducted under their supervision were not successful.

Only much later did I finally understand why my third and fourth patients left (albeit after 300 hours). My supervisors and I really did *not* understand their problems adequately. But more importantly, my response to both patients was critical rather than empathic. Conveying this kind of understanding — as I now believe based on subsequent experiences — would have allowed a successful ending of the analysis of a man with a fairly severe self-disorder. My response to the woman also conveyed criticism. I pathologized her striving for success as a means to bolster her shaky self-esteem. It would have been more helpful to recognize the function her competitiveness had in managing a host of early traumatic experiences. Maybe then this analysis, too, could have come to a successful termination.

In addition to a written examination at the end of my training at the Institute, I was required to write an essay. I thought a lot about my four supervisory experiences and what I learned in each of them. But at the time, I was not ready to set down in writing what I found helpful or unhelpful. At that time, I felt that Joan Fleming had added the most to my learning. She had a discernible but non-intrusive agenda. She created a pleasant atmosphere. She was proud of what we accomplished and asked me to present the termination of the analysis she had supervised at two different seminars. After graduation she also invited me to co-teach the psychoanalytic technique course which I then did for seven years.

The deficits in the supervision I received was a major factor in my involvement with Heinz Kohut. After graduation, in 1964, I sought him out for an extra, fifth supervision — one more than mandatory. I wanted to be a good psychoanalyst, especially clinically good, and although the fifth supervision was time-consuming, expensive and tiring, it proved to be well worth it.

EIGHT ~ Life outside Analysis

When I look back on it, my first decade in Cincinnati was very busy and exciting. In addition to my work at University of Cincinnati College of Medicine, teaching and working in the clinic and in private practice, I was on the staff of the Jewish Hospital, and Holmes Hospital, and — starting in 1957 — psychiatric consultant to the German Consulate in Cleveland while commuting every two weeks to Chicago.

"Psychiatric Consultant to the German Consulate" is an unusual job description for an activity that was very meaningful to me. After an older psychiatrist retired, I was asked to take over the evaluation, diagnosis and recommendation for reparations to Holocaust survivors in our region, who were applying for "restitution" from the German government for their years of slave labor and other suffering under Nazism. I was to determine what "percent" of their mental and physical health had been affected by their experience of incarceration and the losses they suffered.

I think that the one hundred or more survivors I met with between 1957 and 1970 understood without my telling them that I was Jewish myself, and that I would try to help them as much as I could. Many of them asked if we could conduct the interviews in Yiddish, which I understood perfectly well. I have forgotten many of their stories but Anna remembers them because, of course, I told her each one. One man had survived in a closed coffin, with no sunlight for many months, and after the war he was almost blind.

The German government generally accepted whatever "percentage" of injury I indicated. It probably helped that I had graduated from medical school in Heidelberg and understood how the Germans viewed valid medical evidence and psychiatric diagnoses.

Over the same period, I was also the unlikely partner in an early tech start-up. During the late 1950s, I became friendly with a colleague who had come to Cincinnati General Hospital at about the same time as I did. His name was Robert Kalthoff and, for a few years, he was the chief psychiatric resident.

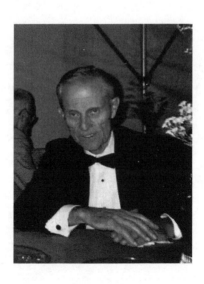

We shared Gottschalk as our training analyst and enjoyed each other's company.

One summer, during Gottschalk's vacation, we decided that we had the time to write a psychiatry textbook based on our experiences at work. Before long, we realized that we needed to find an efficient way to deal with our notes and the medical records we were using. There was a colleague of ours on the psychiatric faculty who was said to have a good system but we looked at it, didn't like it, and decided to develop our own.

Before computers, it was a major problem to keep track of medical records. The issue side-tracked us so completely that we never completed the textbook, but in the process of trying to figure out how to organize, sort and store our files we wound up inventing an early information retrieval system and a machine.

Robert Kalthoff was a very gifted man, a pianist and choral conductor who had studied at the Juilliard School of Music in New York. He was an excellent psychiatrist but like several others who had applied to be candidates at the Chicago Institute, he was for unexplained reasons not accepted. Bob was extremely creative and, in addition, very gifted mechanically. Both he and his brother were good with their hands as well as their minds. We developed the machine that gave birth to the Access Corporation.

In the then pre-computer era, this was an extraordinary idea. Bob found an engineer to translate his idea into a product and, in 1961, began to apply for patents.

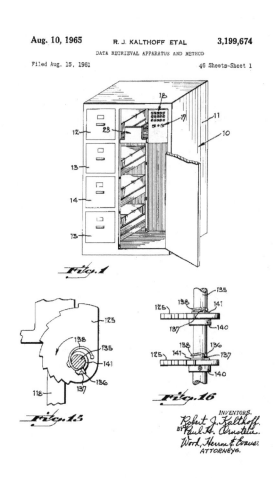

Aug. 10, 1965   R. J. KALTHOFF ETAL   3,199,674

DATA RETRIEVAL APPARATUS AND METHOD

Filed Aug. 15, 1961   46 Sheets-Sheet 1

Fig. 1

Fig. 15

Fig. 16

INVENTORS.
Robert J. Kalthoff.
BY Paul H. Arnolein.
Wood, Herron & Evans.
ATTORNEYS.

Major corporations including Xerox, 3M and GE were interested in acquiring the patents. I thought we'd be rich and immediately went out and bought the complete bound sets of *The International Journal of Psychoanalysis, The Psychoanalytic Quarterly* and *The Journal of the American Psychoanalytic Association*, and bookshelves to hold them.

130

All the corporations decided against buying our product so Bob Kalthoff formed his own company and raised $9 million to start the Access Corporation to manufacture and sell the system. As a co-founder, I was a member of the Board for more than a decade and went to meetings where I learned about business. I learned about how to manage money but then I forgot it all — I didn't have so much money to manage anyhow! I didn't always understand everything that was said at those board meetings but I found it interesting to listen. By 1984, the sales of Access Corporation were $13-14 million and, as a shareholder, I was one of the beneficiaries. I never got rich but it was an extraordinary experience.

At the same time that we enjoyed very busy and fulfilling professional lives, Anna and I were parents of three growing children, who led us further into American culture and whose childhoods were very different from ours.

Both our daughters were lively and outgoing. Miriam was, early on, a writer, who often climbed up into the branch of a tree outside my study and wrote things that she sometimes allowed us to read. As Rafael grew up, he was very popular with girls and boys and played all the ball games boys play in this country. I must confess that I could not join him in these endeavors; Jewish boys in Hajdúnánás did not play ball — they went to *cheder*! But I was very happy to sit on the bleachers and watch. He also turned out to have musical talent and learned to play the piano.

I was surprised by how natural it was for all three of my children to visit their friends' homes after school and to have "sleep-overs" — certainly not what I had done as a child.

I was not a strict father. I tried to be like my father was to me. I remember the unusual time I gave Rafael a slap on the behind because he threw a ball at our garage window and broke it — it seemed deliberately. When I asked him why he had done it, he replied that he was always so good and wanted to do something bad for once.

Anna did most of the parenting. She began her analytic training in 1964, just as I was finishing, and she didn't go to meetings or write much until the mid-1970s. Even then, it didn't take away from her motherliness. We lived ten minutes by car from the hospital and every weekday at noon, she picked up the children from school, drove them home and had lunch with them.

She organized the household to have a system based around a wonderful housekeeper who came in at 7:30 in the morning and left at two, and a series of young women baby-sitters who lived in the top floor of our home rent-free, in exchange for taking care of the children in the afternoons.

Our children, especially Sharone, also led us back to religious observance. I had lost my faith in the Ukraine. When I returned from the labor battalion, I felt that I had nothing to do with God and he had nothing to do with me. The pain I felt had to do with my mother and three siblings who died in Auschwitz. I didn't understand why Jews got stuck in their evolution with a belief in God.

Both Anna and I almost lost the healing and sustaining power of our many Jewish traditions after the war. But my children helped us recapture them. They went to Sunday School and came home with questions. They wanted to hear how we had celebrated our holidays in our homes when we were children.

When our daughter Sharone came home for Seder during her first year in college, she wanted to create a new way for everyone around the table to participate. She asked what freedom meant to each of us. This is when Anna wrote her first Passover story. She spoke about her pre-Shoah experiences often and, whenever the children asked, she would offer snippets of her camp experiences. But they were never a main topic of conversation.

Starting with that Seder and for the next 25 years, Anna wrote and read a story drawn from her experiences in Europe, motivated by a desire to leave a legacy about our destroyed families to our children and grandchildren. These stories became part of our family's *Haggadah*, the Passover story that recounts persecution, slavery and redemption. Those stories have been published in a book called *My Mother's Eyes*.

My children wanted us to attend religious services at the local synagogue. Their friends went to services with their families; they wanted us to go too. I liked to read the Hebrew — I didn't want to lose the language. The nearest synagogue was Reform, and although I didn't like to hear the prayers in English, I enjoyed listening to good sermons.

My own public speaking to large audiences began when I was over 40. From the time I was a resident physician I attended professional meetings to hear senior psychiatrists and psychoanalysts present papers. The first big meeting I attended was the American Psychoanalytic Association meeting in New York City and I attended the annual meeting almost without interruption until 2015. At first, I just listened, then I participated in a number of group discussions and presented papers. I wanted to hear the contributors to the field personally. That helped me to judge whether their writing was worthwhile or not.

You might say I began my professional writing in a very limited way, writing short summaries of Grand Rounds in the Department of Psychiatry at the University of Cincinnati. "I'm going to Grand Rounds," was the, at first, puzzling term I heard when I first came to the United States. I soon learned that it was an old medical tradition that involved the entire departmental staff and other interested people meeting in an auditorium for up to two hours to hear an important speaker. I listened carefully and, since I always liked to write, I wrote up one-page summaries of our Grand Rounds called "Focusing," had them mimeographed, and distributed to about 100 people.

In the late 1950s, I also began writing reviews of books published in German for the *Journal of American Psychiatry*. My first professional paper in English was published in 1961. It was titled "An Experiment in Teaching Psychotherapy to Junior Medical Students" and appeared in the *Journal of Medical Education*. I also co-authored several other papers in the early 1960s.

I never found writing difficult. On the contrary, I enjoyed it. I first began presenting my writing at professional meetings in February of 1967, when Maurice Levine was asked to give a paper at the Ohio Psychiatric Association in Columbus, Ohio and asked me to step in on his behalf. I was honored and very pleased that he trusted me to do it well.

Consequently, at the age of nearly 43, I wrote what I regard as my first important paper, "What Is and What Is Not Psychotherapy?" delineating psychotherapy as distinct from other forms of helpfulness. My English was not an issue by then and I did not worry about the reception I would receive. I thought: if they don't like it, they don't like it. My pride in that paper, even today, has to do with the fact that in it I came close to formulating the self object concept (without this term), before my acquaintance with Heinz Kohut's work on narcissism and self psychology.

On another occasion, some years later, my favorite analytic supervisor, Joan Fleming, asked me to present aspects of my analytic work at her workshop at a Mid-Winter Meeting of the American Psychoanalytic Association. I thought I presented well, much of it "ad-lib." She thought so too. It may have been a compliment she paid me in the middle of my presentation that made me aware of my old anxiety in this setting (with a number of senior analysts present). She asked me what might that be about — as she would have asked in individual supervision.

I told her about my anxiety that I could never emulate my father's ease and eloquence of speaking and I came with that anxiety to this workshop. She stopped me and simply said: "Well, what about now? You just did it!" I began to come home from conferences with the announcement, "Veni, vidi, vici." (I came; I saw; I conquered).

Presenting papers at workshops, seminars and conferences far from Cincinnati became a growing part of my professional life. In 1964, when Rafael, our youngest child, was old enough to travel, I began taking the family to New York and to meetings of the International Psychoanalytic Association.

The IPA met every other year, usually in a European city we were interested in visiting: Vienna, Berlin, Rome, Nice. We had four weeks off every summer and would take these opportunities to meet my father in Europe or in Israel, and to revisit Hungary.

Those were still the years of the Cold War — my

daughter Sharone still remembers the barbed wire, the train conductors at the Austrian border inspecting our passports, and my refusing to acknowledge that I spoke or understood Hungarian. As long as I had friends and relatives living there, I wanted to go back.

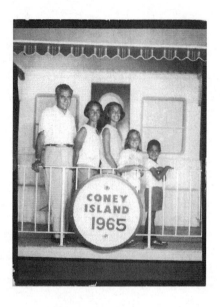

In Budapest, we stayed in a hotel on the Danube from which we could walk everywhere in Pest. I liked to go to bookstores and buy books I couldn't then obtain in the U.S. I also liked to go to the synagogue and listen to sermons in Hungarian. I showed the children the room I lived in at the Rabbinical Seminary and introduced them to the Director who was my old friend.

Some two decades later, I also took a group of my psychoanalytic colleagues on a tour of Budapest. Once again, whenever I wanted to, I pretended not to understand Hungarian. I enjoyed showing my friends around: I took them up to the Castle in Buda; to the Gellért Spa where they took the waters; to a nice restaurant on the Danube. I called a friend of mine from rabbinical school who had remained in Hungary to get us tickets to the Opera. He did and we all went — nearly 20 of us.

As a teenager, my friends and I always climbed up to the last cheapest seats in the house after standing in line for tickets for hours in the cold. Suddenly at the Opera with these analysts, I realized all we had missed downstairs. I had never sat in the orchestra before.

I enjoyed going back on my own terms.

NINE ~ Kohut

During my years in Cincinnati and now, for the past 15 years in Boston, four pictures have hung on a wall in my study.

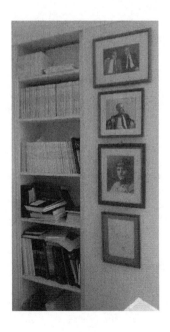

On top is an impressive, life-like image of Heinz Kohut

with his right arm on my shoulders; beneath it, Levine's gently smiling image; beneath that, my father in his World War I Austro-Hungarian lieutenant's uniform; then a pencil-drawn profile of Michael Balint with his ironic smile.

These are the four men who had the most formative influence on my psychoanalytic development, steadily looking at me as I work.

I first met Heinz Kohut during my first two years of training at the Chicago Institute. He taught a two-year theory course on Freud and ego psychology and it was a dazzling performance. Without notes, he gave a coherent lecture for up to two hours that was so well constructed that it could have been put directly into print. I admired and envied his brilliant exposition and detailed knowledge of Freud. He could present Freud's ideas thoroughly and as though there were no contradictions or difficulties in them; as if all fitted well together.

His pedagogy, on the other hand, was dreadful. He spoke without allowing any questions or leaving time for discussion. One of us was assigned to take notes, which he would read at the beginning of the next session. Two weeks later, when we started the session with our questions, they seemed "cold," but Kohut wove his new lecture around those questions. There was no real give and take and that interfered with my learning.

However, Heinz Kohut proved to be a very different kind of teacher when he substituted for Maxwell Gitelson at the termination seminar that we took as fifth-year candidates. Gitelson (later President of the International Psychoanalytic Association) was not a pleasant seminar leader. After we presented terminated analyses, Gitelson's comments would be generally interesting in terms of his (sometimes quite rigid) ego psychological perspective. But at the end he almost always said, "This was good psychotherapy but not an analysis." I wondered what they had been teaching us for five years if none of the presenters had been able to conduct a successful analysis! Had our teachers reflected on their way of teaching sufficiently? I knew Joan Fleming and Theresa Benedek had studied supervision and written a book about it. Were the others on the faculty conversant with or affected by their ideas? Gitelson certainly did not seem to be.

When Gitelson was unable to be present, usually Kohut substituted for him. He always found something worthwhile to pick out of the presentation. He would then elaborate on it respectfully, appreciating the student-analyst's efforts, even when not always successful. He used the opportunity, even at that late stage, to teach and not to judge. He created a climate of learning and was able to correct details of the analyst's approach in a manner that did not shame the presenter, but enriched the clinical data for the analyst as well as for the class. Still another feature of Kohut's teaching stood out for me: he moved from the clinical to the theoretical and from the theoretical to the clinical with ease. He never imposed the theory on the data but moved seamlessly from the data to theory.

It was mainly this very last feature that I most admired in Kohut's approach, in addition to his obvious *humanity* in clinical supervision. I very much wanted to benefit from this particular feature of his clinical teaching in my postgraduate years. Up until this time none of us had any idea that Kohut had original ideas of his own that would be different from Freud's and Hartmann's ego psychology and structural theory. We were all impressed with his synthesis and integration of these theories into a coherent (American) "main-street" psychoanalysis of its time.

Until then, Balint had been my model of a clinician but, in those sessions of the termination seminar that he taught, Kohut surpassed him. You might call my attitude towards him idealization — some of my friends teased me about idealizing Kohut in a mildly sarcastic manner — but I had and have a different view of it. Idealization is a form of appreciation: you feel enriched by a person's contribution to your own learning or understanding. Idealizing Kohut did not, for me, mean exaggerating his talents and the importance of his ideas. I felt that he fully deserved my admiration.

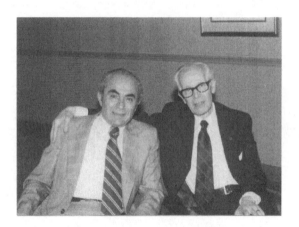

I decided that the best way to learn about Kohut's clinical approach was to seek supervision with him, even though I had completed my four required, supervised analyses. He did not have a faculty appointment apart from the one at the Chicago Institute but had a private practice.

I brought the clinical evaluation of a new patient to my first appointment and was greatly surprised that my diagnosis of a complex neurosis was questioned by Kohut. The patient, in his mid-twenties, single, intelligent, well-spoken, tall, handsome, carefully dressed, was a troubled young psychiatric resident. He showed some unusual symptoms and behavior patterns in the area of self-regulation, which Kohut attributed to his "narcissistic disorder," rather then to a straightforward neurosis. He added that the sort of problem the patient presented was in all likelihood more complicated than a neurosis — "but let's wait and see what you find in the analysis as you proceed." He implied that I should discover the nature of the patient's problems from our experience with each other.

My patient was constantly restless, could not sit still, could not read alone in his room for any length of time, got easily bored. He had a little black book with the telephone numbers of women ready to receive him whenever he called.

At one point, Kohut suggested in connection with one of the patient's compulsive habits that he would tell Mr. I. something like this: when he had to run around the block (even in the middle of his working day) several times or rush home to take a cold shower, he was attempting to stir himself up, to revitalize himself. And when he needed hot showers or to have intercourse on demand with one of his many girlfriends (day or night), he was trying to calm himself. My response was that I could not say this to Mr. I. Kohut wondered why? Well, it does not sound to me like an analytic intervention, I said. OK, Kohut replied calmly. "If that is how you feel, do not say it."

During the week that followed, these kinds of issues again dominated the sessions and, against some inner resistance, I found myself telling Mr. I. just what Kohut suggested, that he was trying to self-regulate.

To my amazement, my patient visibly relaxed and said, "That's true, where did you get that? Nobody has ever told me that before." With Kohut's help I hit upon the *function* these compulsive behaviors served for Mr. I. With that statement, I let him know that what he felt compelled to do had a purpose; a definite function. What I learned was that Kohut's suggestion provided a meaningful *analytic intervention* with salutary consequences for the analytic process.

As this analysis proceeded I presented more, many (to me) puzzling problems to Kohut. He was, in 1966, working on the manuscript of his first book, *The Analysis of the Self.* From time to time, as I told him about a problem I was experiencing, he would open his drawer, pull out a page and say that he had just written something for his book about the experience I was reporting. After a few such episodes, I asked him if I might read the entire manuscript. His answer was a gem I still cherish: "no, *let the patient teach you how to analyze him.*"

This kind of supervision helped me acquire my knowledge of self psychology directly from the analytic treatment process. This also had for me the felicitous consequence of recognizing early on how tightly the method of observation (empathy, i.e., vicarious introspection) and data (the nature of a patient's problems) as well as the process of change ("cure") were inseparably connected. Slowly, I began to understand how empathy, coupled with a theory that guides the analyst to the patient's inner world, are essential requirements of a useful theory for psychoanalytic treatment. I later learned from other patients more precisely how my subjectivity played a decisive role in the treatment process. That essentially led to a "*disciplined subjectivity*." Without a good guiding theory we can only go so far in any psychoanalytic treatment.

Learning from patients is a life-long blessing in our profession — if we are open to it. Such openness is what I feel I have gained from Kohut's work.

It is in the course of this supervisory experience and of having acquired extensive knowledge in self psychology that I could finally understand why two of my four supervised analytic patients left their treatment with me without "proper" termination. My third patient felt misunderstood or simply not understood regarding his compulsive extramarital relations. Even the use of the word "compulsive" (though he used it first, with considerable shame) put his behavior into the category of pathology, although I knew that it was the only way he could have sexual pleasure. He heard it as my wanting him to give it up, to stop it. Only later could I reflect on the fact that had I been able to speak with him about the *function* that his behavior served for him, had I really been able to look at this need from *his* perspective, we might have been able to work together more fruitfully and terminate the analysis successfully.

With my fourth patient a similar problem came to the fore. Had I been able to see what my supervisor considered "penis-envy," in a different light — as I learned from Kohut — this analysis might also have ended more successfully, with mutual consent. I might have been able to recognize the patient's ambition for accomplishment and also realize that her shaky self-esteem had to be bolstered with many of her behaviors. She might then have felt that I was on her side; that I understood her predicament from

145

within her own perspective and could have appreciated her sustained effort to remedy it.

These two analyses demanded a sustained, empathic immersion in the patient's experiences to lead me to the view from within their inner world. Self psychology gave me a broader view of the human condition: *a view of human experience from within,* and not the impersonal dynamics of a mental apparatus.

There are many fundamental differences between traditional ego psychology and self psychology which were, at first, difficult for me to absorb. Based on his clinical observations, Kohut questioned the primacy of the sexual and aggressive drives as motivating psychological development and psychopathology. Instead, he considered the child's emotional environment as being potentially pathogenic if it failed to provide developmentally requisite validating responses and merger experiences with the caretakers' idealized strength. Critics considered these ideas as not psychoanalytic because only drive-related unconscious fantasies have been viewed as "truly psychoanalytic." Kohut was dismissed as being an "environmentalist."

Another important difference between the two theories is related to Kohut's views on Narcissism. Traditional psychoanalytic theory considered patients who suffered from Narcissistic Personality and Behavior Disorders as unanalyzable. Describing the various narcissistic (later called self object) transferences offered these patients the possibility of undergoing psychoanalysis. In a sense, Kohut undid the pejorative attitude regarding narcissistic disturbances that had characterized the profession — and still does in many quarters.

After my supervision, from 1969 to 1981, I became a member of a small group Kohut organized to read and discuss his manuscript of *The Analysis of the Self* before it was published. It included Arnold Goldberg, one of my best friends. Anna and I always stayed with Arnold and Connie Goldberg when we slept overnight in Chicago. We were also close to Paul and Marion Tolpin and to Michael Basch, who was considered the most brilliant of the group and died young, of a brain tumor. Other members of the group included Robert Stolorow, Bernard Brandchaft, and Art Malin who flew to Chicago from Los Angeles every other Saturday for our meetings. There were also members in Canada, one in Paris and one in Rome. These meetings provided significant learning experiences and the basis for life-long friendships.

My long introductions to the two volumes of Kohut's collected work, *The Search for the Self: Selected Writings of Heinz Kohut*, are the most comprehensive statements I can make about his importance. Here, I will only point out that Kohut didn't seem radical or controversial to me, even though at the Chicago Institute, two of his colleagues did not even regard him as an acceptable member of the analytic faculty. He was well liked personally and was friendly with the rest of the faculty and candidates.

I somehow *knew* that the mainstream was old-fashioned. The majority of analysts worshipped Freud and relied on what seemed to me a doctrinaire approach to patients. Kohut just seemed to have a newer outlook. My chief, Maurice Levine, thought we should invite him to Cincinnati. But by the time Kohut came for the first time, Levine was hospitalized. I persuaded some of the other Cincinnati faculty to invite him.

He would fly in on Friday nights and present on

Saturdays and was always well received. On Saturday afternoons, he and I often went for a walk and one Saturday, he suddenly stopped and said to me, "You might be wondering about my Jewishness. My father was Jewish — my mother is not." Actually, both his parents were Jewish but his mother converted later in her life. Later I heard that his father walked to synagogue in the manner of observant Jews but that his mother drove and got out of the car a few blocks away from the synagogue.

I didn't discuss Judaism with Kohut. I knew he had been born in Vienna in 1913, and had fled after 1938. I also knew that he was not accepting of his Jewishness. Once I was having lunch in a deli with Kohut and his son. He ordered a ham and cheese sandwich and made a fuss when he could not get it. I didn't like his rejection of Jewish identity but I thought: who am I to demand he be exactly the way I would like him to be? It was none of my business. I got what I needed from him.

I wanted Anna to have the same extraordinary experience I was having with Kohut. We already knew that studying together, we could more quickly digest what we were learning. But by the 1970s, we came to realize that we lived in a largely reactionary psychoanalytic environment in Cincinnati. Very few colleagues shared our deep interest in Balint or in Kohut.

My department was classically oriented. Six of us had lunch most days of the week: a clinical psychologist, a social worker, and the rest psychiatrists. I expressed my enthusiasm for Kohut's ideas and shared my own experiences, but I didn't argue with my colleagues or minimize their ways of working.

We got along very well. I spoke out when I disagreed

with them but didn't feel I had to train them or win them over to my way of thinking. Therefore, our friendships lasted until we left Cincinnati.

Although we resided in Cincinnati, our intellectual life in psychoanalysis was lived in other places. Anna and I provided one another with the mutual emotional and intellectual support required to live in what we thought of as Cincinnati's psychoanalytic desert.

I had begun teaching psychoanalysis at the Chicago Institute just after I graduated in 1964. When a group of the people who had been commuting to Chicago from Cincinnati decided to establish an institute of our own to serve the tri-state area of Ohio, Kentucky and Indiana, I was involved. It took two years to work out the curriculum. I wanted to teach the psychoanalytic process, integrating Kohut's self psychology with Freud's ego psychology.

I became a training analyst and a supervisor at the Cincinnati Institute right away, but Anna was not accepted as a training analyst for 20 years. They had nothing against her but we were seen as two strong powerful people and the five or six other senior analysts seemed to feel that one Ornstein was enough! As Kohutians, we were considered outside of the psychoanalytic mainstream.

For many years I was the only self psychologist who was a member of the Center for Advanced Psychoanalytic Studies at Princeton. Our group of senior analysts was made up of colleagues who had a different psychoanalytic orientation. They often teased me about my theory but they never got to me. I could always contradict them. They could not even understand my perspective. I liked them as people but I thought they were not forward-looking. I was so clear about my own ideas that I didn't find their opposition a problem. I could test out my ideas with my wife.

In the mid-1970s, we developed an international Center for the Study of Psychoanalytic Self Psychology within the Department of Psychiatry and were able to attract students. We had clinicians visit the University of Cincinnati and stay for anywhere from a few months to two years.

While still in supervision with Kohut, I had begun to assemble his writings prior to his work on narcissism and self psychology; my aim was to trace the precursors of his new ideas and the project took two decades. I read through all of his published and unpublished papers as well as the proceedings of discussions not meant for publication. I put them in chronological sequence, edited and introduced them. The first covered his work from 1950 to 1978; the second, from 1978 to 1981. The first volume was published in 1978; he did not live to see the second, which was published in 1991. My very long introductions attest to my belief in the importance of Kohut's ideas.

Heinz Kohut died of heart failure in 1981, at the age of 68, after delivering a talk at the Berkeley Self Psychology Conference "On Empathy." We felt the loss acutely. But he left us the broad outlines of a systematic approach to self psychology, and many specific details were worked out later by his students, published or transmitted in lectures and supervision to the next generation. They established what is now called the *International Journal of Psychoanalytic Self Psychology* and held annual meetings.

When Kohut received invitations to speak abroad in the late 1970s, he often suggested that Anna and I speak in his place. We began to travel internationally to teach self psychology and, in 1983, Anna and I began giving yearly workshops in Konstanz, Germany. The participating analysts presented cases to us and we discussed them. I enjoyed focusing on what they had difficulty understanding and helping them. The Germans we met were mostly younger than we were. We also introduced self psychology to Austria and Israel. Another organization we worked with was the New England Educational Institute which ran continuing education programs for professionals in Cape Cod and in the Berkshires during the summer.

The initial resistance to Kohut's ideas in the so-called mainstream of psychoanalysis slowly changed. At first, self psychology was taught in a few courses in some institutes under the label of "deviant schools." This gave way to the label "alternative school." However, this ecumenism appears to be only skin-deep in many places. True legitimacy of self psychology in the eyes of the majority is still a long way off, requiring a better understanding of what psychoanalysis is, how to relate the analyst's subjectivity to his or her guiding theory and practice.

During the 1990s and the 2000s, Anna and I introduced self psychology to many other countries. We conducted more than two hundred seminars and workshops not only in Europe but in South America, Turkey, and as far away as Bali. Self psychology has become in many respects very different since Kohut's death — we might even speak now of many *self psychologies* — perhaps not all of them of equal value; time will tell. His theory and treatment principles opened up a creative reservoir: many analysts and psychotherapists all over the world expanded and modified what Kohut left behind.

We now live in a pluralistic world in psychoanalysis, which was ushered in (in the U.S.) by Kohut's pioneering work and threatened the dominance of ego psychology.

My own contributions, together with Anna, focused on microscopic and macroscopic features of the psychoanalytic treatment process. When I was invited to give the Plenary Presentation at the annual meeting of the American Psychoanalytic Association in May of 2002, I spoke of *"The Elusive Concept of the Psychoanalytic Process."* In it I recounted my focus on this issue throughout my professional life. I stressed that the microprocess (the moment to moment interaction) was dominated by the analyst's subjectivity; whereas the macroprocess was guided by the analyst's particular theory. Every analytic process will inevitably be punctuated by a variety of entanglements between patient and analyst. Whatever these entanglements might be about, the two participants will have to find their idiosyncratic ways to disentangle them. The analyst's particular guiding theory can only offer general principles for their resolution.

Seeing patients, supervising, writing and teaching psychoanalysis gave me a unique opportunity never to stand still, even while in my office with my patients. In fact, there was a steady demand for adjusting and adapting to the needs of each unique personality. Travel enabled me to learn from the various ways in which people in different countries think about and practice psychoanalysis. It was a humbling experience that repeatedly raised the question: what is psychoanalysis?

Psychoanalysis is more than a profession, and more than a set of ideas to aid us in the healing of the mental anguish and pain that create problems in living. It is a view of the world and of the self in depth. We cannot put on and take off our special "theoretical glasses" at will to see the inner world of our patients. These "glasses" become a part of us. We acquire a specific psychoanalytic view of the human condition mainly through the psychoanalytic transformations in our own selves. We can and should be ready to change our theories as new experiences demand it. However, these changes have to go hand in hand with a requisite internal change. Otherwise these remain a "mere technique" and not an emotionally meaningful part of a human interaction in which our "professional self" has to participate as fully as possible.

At various intervals, ongoing clinical experience demanded that I redefine my understanding of what psychoanalysis was. I realized that there were problems within me, in relation to particular patient's needs and demands that I could not properly respond to. This never-ending reflection on what we do as analysts and how we do it is one of the incomparable rewards of our lives in psychoanalysis.

TEN ~ Retirement and Family

I didn't know that all three of my children would grow up to become psychiatrists, that two of them would marry psychiatrists, and that two would even become psychoanalysts! I thought it was a good idea for my children to go into medicine, but it wasn't something I felt they absolutely had to do. However, by the time they were teenagers, Rafael and Sharone decided that they wanted to go to medical school, and I don't remember any difficulties they had in that regard that I got involved in. Miriam had a different kind of psyche and was searching for a long time, deciding what she should do with her life.

I never had that kind of situation in my own life so I had to learn how to respond to her. She graduated from the University of Michigan, went to Boston and worked for about a year in a bagel bakery and a pizza shop. There, she was a labor organizer who dared to demand better pay for the workers. I was aware that she didn't know what she wanted, and didn't understand why she had to do this, that, and the other. Finally during a long car drive to Boston in September of 1980, we had a deeper conversation and, afterwards, I wrote her a long letter.

I wanted her to feel loved. And I wanted to tell her that I was not going to interfere, but I understood that she was a little bit lost. It turned out that my letter was very important to her. She kept it and, since I myself no longer remember exactly what I wrote, she suggested that I include some excerpts as a sample of my parenting.

Dearest Gyöngybogárkám, I began with a Hungarian endearment that can best be translated as Dear Pearl-bug.

Yom Kippur always makes me think of my family... So on this Yom Kippur, I remembered you sitting in your new car, comfortably, self-assuredly, driving toward a definite destination. The thought came to me about the many exits in the road that could be taken. All of them, I thought, could lead to interesting and worthwhile destinations —with the option of returning to the "main highway" if one felt side-tracked, as we did for a while when looking for gasoline. Remember, we couldn't find any gas despite urgently and restlessly searching. So we decided to go back onto the highway anyhow, hoping that we could find some. And we did.

This could almost be put into the form of a Hasidic story.

If you go on a journey, focus relaxedly on the going! If you focus on the search of just one specific destination, this will impede your journey because you will always have to wonder (sometimes even obsessively): which way should I turn? Did I miss the right turn? Where is it? and often, in desperation, "What am I looking for anyhow?"

But if you travel with the focus on traveling itself (life as it is), on the opportunities to take in the scenery with all of its landmarks — animate and inanimate — and if you pause to get acquainted with whatever strikes you as beautiful, interesting, enriching, horizon-enlarging, perspective-building, etc — the destination, your evolving destination, will be the natural outcome of your journey.

You have had from Day One in your life what it takes to have a meaningful and safe journey... So when you went to Boston after graduation "to find yourself" we did not view it a priori as getting off the highway but as taking a side trip through the scenic route. You wanted to find out first-hand what another way of life looked like.

We became concerned only when you expressed concern that you felt side-tracked and when you had to exclude or could no longer include in your life the intellectual, aesthetic and literary interests that you had until then. But even that seemed of little concern, until you expressed the feeling that you were nowhere, that you lost what had always sparked a flame in you (and made you capable of sparking it in others with whom you came into contact.)

I think that our mentality — Mom's and mine — our need to have both feet on the ground even while dreaming, our need to stay on the main road and keep advancing, our need not to allow ourselves to be side-tracked, based on our life experiences and temperament may have been — among other things — hampering our children in their journey — especially in feeling that the journey they are on was indeed their journey. After all, your temperament, your life experiences, and your talents safeguard a wider latitude for travel. You would therefore have to have a different journey.

The main point is this: you can't lose the road permanently. What you gained thus far is yours to keep.

The punchline of my Hassidic story is this: one is thrust into this world in a way that one can only find out where one is going while already on the trip. The destination can only appear on the horizon if you let yourself in for a surprise. You can change course mid-stream anytime. Even after completing a segment of a trip you can take another — the idea is that we are constantly on the road if we just recognize and take advantage of it.

Ever since Adam and Eve left paradise, we were not given the chance to wait until we are ready to leave for a journey. We are on a perpetual traveling schedule and cannot get off it.

With much love,

Father

I remember that writing this letter came very easily to me. I knew that Miriam would find her way. After that, she worked for two years with sexually-abused children. I thought that experience would lead her to psychiatry, as it eventually did.

Looking back at it at the age of 91, if I had to do it all over again, I would spend more time with my children. They deserved more of my attention. I was a traditional father, preoccupied by my work, usually in my study with my books, the kind of father that was taken for granted in American culture of the 1950s and 1960s. My old friend Steve Hornstein was, I think, more or less the same. Part of the reason was our European tradition; part of it was that I was bent on professional accomplishment. I loved very much what I was doing. I wanted to climb the academic ladder and to become not just a good, but an extraordinary analyst. I didn't do what my son Rafael would do when he had children 40 years later — to postpone some professional things to be a better father.

Anna did most of the parenting when our children were

small. When it came time for them to choose colleges, I talked with them a little about where they wanted to go but not very much. Sharone had been a toddler when we lived in Waltham, Massachusetts. We had pushed her stroller through the Brandeis campus when it was still being built and joked that one day she would go to college there. She did! Miriam chose the University of Michigan; and Rafael, Wesleyan. But the fact is I didn't really know what distinguished one college from another — I trusted that they knew.

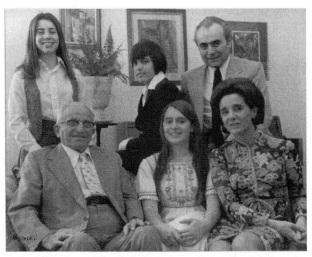

The Ornsteins in Cincinnati with Lajos Ornstein, circa 1973

I drove Sharone to Brandeis. She went into her dormitory and started talking to people and I became aware that I was suddenly no longer needed. I cried when I left her dormitory, but I am well known for becoming emotional. I went to visit friends in Boston that evening and there, I began to hiccup. My hiccups lasted for three days and I knew that it must have been related to separation from my daughter.

It happened again when I took Miriam to school in Ann Arbor but, interestingly, not when I took Rafael to Wesleyan, and it has never happened since. I realized that children have to leave the family but, somehow, letting go of my daughters provoked a different inner response from me than letting go of my son. I maintained a very significant relation with Rafael but apparently it was different.

All three of my children came back to Cincinnati to attend medical school. Because Anna and I were professors there, Sharone studied free-of-charge, Miriam had to pay something and Rafael a little more. But they did not live at home and had their own lives. Most of the time, they had relationships with people I liked. When there was someone I found objectionable, I was outspoken. I said something like "that's an impossible character." But most of the time, I think I was accepting. I was 15 when I myself left home for Budapest. The first two summers, I went home but after that I didn't. I never thought about it but, in retrospect, part of my attitude towards my children felt natural. Part of it was that I must have been taking on my father's way of allowing me to find my own way of living and being.

I didn't worry too much about whom my children would marry. I listened to what they told me and trusted that, ultimately, they would make the right decisions and be satisfied with their lives. It was important to me that they marry Jews and they all did, without it ever being discussed.

The first one to marry was Sharone. She met Jeff

Halpern, the man who was to become her husband, in New York City, at a psychiatry department party when Sharone had just finished her training and Jeff was a resident. We were still living in Cincinnati, so it took time to get to know him. I came to admire my son-in-law very much.

Miriam and Rafael had more romantic attachments because they did not marry when they were younger, like Sharone. I didn't meet all of them and I know I probably would not have liked all of them. Luckily, we were living far away. Only when we moved to Boston did we learn more about their lives. They both married people whom we love: Rafael married a child psychiatrist, Susannah Sherry. Miriam married a musician, Joe Reid, who had two children from an earlier marriage.

So I have seven grandchildren: Zachary and Noah Halpern; Benjamin and Sarah Reid; Adina, Nicholas and Jeremy Ornstein. I love to listen to what they are thinking and doing.

In 2000, at the age of 76, I retired from the University of Cincinnati Medical School. After so many years of analyzing, supervising, writing, learning and teaching, I felt that I finally knew how to do analysis, and it was hard to give up. If it had been possible, I would have liked to have been able to continue practicing every day from 8 to 10 in the morning, and then spending the rest of time reading and writing. But Kafka and Dostoyevsky were waiting for me; I wanted to read, think and write about them.

It took me two more years to wind down my private practice and to stop supervision. In 2000, we sold the house in which we had lived since 1959, and moved to Boston to be closer to our children and grandchildren.

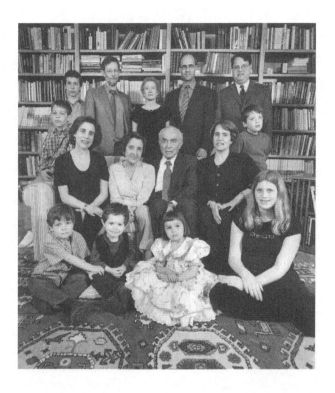

I was not expecting to do any more supervision but when we got there, two advanced psychoanalytic candidates who heard about our arrival called me up and asked for it. I supervised one for three years and the other for one. It gave me yet another opportunity to learn, and I found that I still enjoyed the interaction.

But finally I had time to read. I had begun to read Dostoyevsky in America — I had not read him in Budapest. Anna and I started listening to an audio version of *Notes from Underground* in the car, during our long trips between

Cincinnati and Cape Cod to give workshops, and I knew I wanted to write about him.

I read Tolstoy too, but he didn't grab me in the same way and I was not interested in writing about his work. Anna Karenina doesn't seem as deep to me as the brothers Karamazov or others among Dostoyevsky's characters. Dostoyevsky gets me so involved that I read and reread his work without losing interest. I'm fascinated by the power of the author's language, imagery, and insights. I've now read all of Dostoyevsky's writing — in chronological order. I'm struck by the fact that — just like many of my patients — he never changes the subject!

I began leading study groups of Dostoyevsky's work with Anna at the annual meetings of the American Psychoanalytic every January, and I continued for ten years. In a way, I was doing what Zvi Goldberg had done at the Rabbinical Seminary in Budapest with the writings of Freud, Reik and Ferenczi.

I asked the group members: did they read the entire novel? Only parts? How did they feel while reading? Sampling the readers' subjective reactions often helps understand how we read and interpret Dostoyevsky.

The Russian master's literary productions are a goldmine for psychoanalysts. He was a depth-psychologist par excellence — one might say he was a psychoanalyst before Freud, a daring, unsparing explorer of his own psyche and therefore unusually capable of describing the inner world of his characters. Progressing chronologically in his work, the characters grow, deepen and become ever more complex, culminating in *The Brothers Karamazov*. I published a long article summarizing my thoughts on Dostoyevsky in America Imago in 2012.

The year 2016 will be the first year that I don't go to the annual meeting of American psychoanalysts. When the time comes to stop traveling, you have to accept it. Will I miss it? I don't think of it in those terms. I did enough of it.

I'm very lucky to have had a very long life and, with the exception of the six months in 1944, enjoyed almost every minute of it. I'm actually surprised that I'm still alive.

When we first came to the United States, I was diagnosed with pulmonary fibrosis (scarring of the lungs) but for 60 years, I was asymptomatic. Then, while I was at work in my hospital in Cincinnati in the 1980s, I had a heart attack. I walked by myself to the Emergency Room. Then, on my way to a speaking engagement in Minneapolis in 2001, I collapsed on the way to the airplane. Cardiac arrest. Two ladies who happened to be nurses gave me mouth-to-mouth resuscitation before a defibrillator was located and used to save my life.

In the summer in 2013, while flying back to Boston from Cincinnati, I developed a bronchitis that activated the pulmonary fibrosis and interfered with the flow of oxygen to my brain. Since that bronchitis, I can no longer recollect many things that I could remember before. Only then did I stop writing. I was 88.

I have difficulty remembering names when I need them and then, sometimes a day or two later, they come to my mind without my trying to bring them into awareness. Dates are almost entirely gone from my memory, but sometimes I can recall an event from long ago in extraordinary detail.

When I read (in English, Hungarian, and German), I understand everything but it doesn't stick. I enjoy it but I don't retain it. It's annoying but I reread certain chapters again and again because the enjoyment is still present. To take pleasure in reading is a great gift.

I also enjoy watching television: a must for me is Fareed Zakaria on Sundays. But it bothers me that hearing people over the telephone is sometimes a problem. Every morning, however, I check my email. I have no problem using a computer. I get a lot of email from friends all over the world. I have a friend in Germany who, every week, sends me the entire *Süddeutsche Zeitung* and I go through every page in German. It lets me know what's going on in Europe, especially in Hungary. Friends often send me clippings from the *Jerusalem Post* and *Ha'aretz* that I read. And I have the *New York Times* delivered to my door every day and read it along with my breakfast.

No one else in my family lived as long as I have, except my maternal grandfather who was 96 when he died on the way to Auschwitz. My mother wasn't even 50; my brothers and my sister, not even 20. My father was 78 when he died in Israel. Lusia Hornstein was the first of our group in Heidelberg to die. She was only 71 and it was losing someone who was like part of my family. Steve Hornstein contracted Alzheimer's disease even before that. He died at 83, in 2008.

It was a very difficult experience for me to see my oldest friend slowly developing Alzheimer's disease. Steve made the diagnosis himself while we were still in Cincinnati. He retired from doing surgery soon after an incident where he forgot where he was downtown. After Lusia died in 1998, he left Cincinnati to live in an apartment near his son and daughter in Minnesota. As long as he could travel, he visited us in Boston when he visited his oldest son. I took him with me on my various travels in town — to get a haircut or to go grocery shopping. He no longer enjoyed museums. I had to converse with him about his difficulties gently as his difficulty increased. I did not talk with him on the phone — because he would speak slowly and it was difficult for me to hear him. Having experienced his very slow decline, his death was a relief for his family and for me and my family.

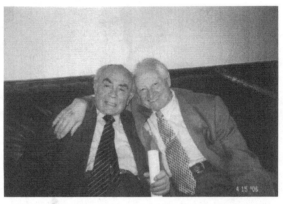

Lifelong friends Paul Ornstein (left) and Steve Hornstein

I haven't given up living yet. I still enjoy waking up every day to Anna's breakfast and the newspaper. I wouldn't mind living to 100 so long as I could continue to read and enjoy my family! Luckily I have never experienced any physical pain from my illness. My strength at this age is that I have Anna with me. We were married when she was 19 and I was 22. Now she is 88 and I am 91. If you live this long, it doesn't depend only on you, but on how you've been living all along and with whom.

I have never said it out loud, but most important in my life have been my wife and my children, even more than psychoanalysis. If you understand them and respond to them — that's the most important thing and I feel I had it. I have enjoyed my summer, and hope that, now in the fall, there is more life.

October 2015

AFTERWORD ~ Hungary in 1940-1945

by Charles Fenyvesi

I was born in 1937 in Debrecen, 29 miles from Hajdúnánás, where the Ornstein family lived. Members of my family shared some of Paul Ornstein's experiences of the war years. But my mother decided to move to Budapest equipped with birth certificates certifying that we were Christians. Since then, as a journalist and author, I have been often called upon to explain the unusual situation of Jews in Hungary during the Second World War.

Hitler's war officially began on September 1, 1939, with the German invasion of Poland. It did not spill over to Hungary until November of 1941 when Budapest joined the Berlin-Tokyo Axis. Then, Hungary agreed to dispatch more than half a million men to fight the Soviet Union, and passed a law prohibiting Jews to serve in the military.

However, head of state Miklós Horthy resisted German pressures to isolate in ghettos the country's more than 800,000 Jews. (That number included some 100,000 Christians of Jewish origin, whom the new Hungarian legislation, following the Nazi pattern, counted as members of the Jewish race.) Horthy also refused to deport to the Reich Hungarian citizens to what the Germans claimed

169

were "work camps." Instead, the Hungarian parliament set up an alternative for Jews and other "political unreliables," such as Social Democrats and Communists, known as Labor Service units (*Munkaszolgálat,* sometimes translated as Labor Battalions), compulsory for all able-bodied Jewish males from age 18 to 55. A typical assignment was hand-digging trenches to trap Russian tanks. The conscripts worked long hours and their guards beat them severely at the slightest pretext — or no pretext at all.

Horthy acknowledged that he was "an old-fashioned social anti-semite" though he played cards once a week with the country's wealthiest Jews. He made no secret of his objections to Nazi policies and to killing Jews. As a result of his sentiments, Hungary would retain Europe's last intact large Jewish community, though Jews came under the pressure of regulations limiting their movements and expropriating their wealth. Earning a living became exceedingly difficult.

In the spring of 1942, the Nazis controlled most of the continent and Adolf Hitler's boast of making Europe *Judenrein* seemed a realistic option. The great majority of Poland's three and a half million Jews had already been shot or incinerated and sealed wagons were now ferrying members of smaller Jewish communities to Auschwitz and other death camps. Anglo-American forces had landed in Italy, but Allied advances in the Soviet Union and North Africa seemed excruciatingly slow, while the huge network of Nazi concrete fortifications along the Atlantic shore were reinforced around the clock.

Beginning to sniff the wind of an Allied victory, however, in March of 1942, Horthy appointed as Prime Minister Miklós Kállay, from one of the country's oldest families. Kállay also had many Jewish friends, many of them from the northeastern region where the Ornsteins and my extended family lived and prospered. He cunningly insisted that the answer to "the Jewish question" had to wait until after the war's end. What he would not reveal publicly was his certainty of an eventual German defeat. He engaged in secret talks with the Allies in the hope of negotiating a separate peace. Jewish leaders — as well as anti-Nazi Gentiles — had little doubt whose side he favored.

After two years of Kállay's dodging German demands, Hitler lost patience. On March 19, 1944, when Paul Ornstein was in his last year of rabbinical school in Budapest, Wehrmacht tanks rolled into Hungary, occupying a nominal ally. The German ambassador in Budapest summoned Kállay who secured temporary, political asylum at the embassy of neutral Turkey. His replacement was an avowed Nazi, Döme Sztójay. Starting April 5, 1944, Jews were obliged to wear a yellow Star of David. Between May 15 and July 8, Hungary's virulently anti-semitic gendarmerie proudly reported that its men administered the deportation of 434,351 Jews in 147 trains. During those months, cattle wagons crammed with Jews left Hungary for Auschwitz. Only after the Pope and the Swedish king warned of dire consequences for Hungary in a post-war settlement, did Horthy stop the trains.

In June the Allies landed in Normandy and the Red Army advanced toward Hungary from the east. That fall, Horthy finally took the step he had long contemplated. In a radio address to his nation on October 15, 1944 (as Paul Ornstein describes in his memoir) Horthy declared Hungary's neutrality and ordered units fighting the Soviets to lay down their arms. The Germans canceled both projects and installed in power their local auxiliaries, the fanatically anti-semitic Arrow Cross. Horthy was placed under house arrest in a German castle and Kállay was sent to the Dachau concentration camp. Once again, the trains to Auschwitz began running, crowded with Hungarian Jews "like sardines in a tin." In charge was Adolf Eichmann, the SS expert in implementing the Final Solution. Arrow Cross members gleefully assisted.

Gentile friends and impeccable Christian birth certificates saved some members of my extended family. But my grandmother Róza, 72, and others of her generation turned down such offers and followed the government's orders to report at the train stations.

My father and my mother's three brothers were lucky enough to survive the Labor Service, but my wife's uncle perished in the copper mine Bor in German-occupied Yugoslavia where working and living conditions were so inhuman that only a few men were able to return home after the fighting stopped.

Treatment of the Jewish conscripts, most of them attached to Hungarian military units on the Russian front, depended on their Gentile commanders and guards, some of them sadists. One such Hungarian officer proudly proclaimed: "No Jews will return home from here." On the other hand, other officers, probably the minority, were decent human beings — one of them Minister of Defense Vilmos Nagybaczoni-Nagy who went out of his way when visiting the troops to warn that no one in a Labor Service unit could be mistreated. (The Germans insisted that he be fired and arrested him. In 1965, Yad Vashem honored him as a Righteous Gentile.)

Jews were also at risk if captured by the Soviet enemy. The Red Army did not distinguish between Labor Service conscripts and regular Hungarian soldiers. Both groups of prisoners of war were dispatched to do forced labor in the Gulag. The number of casualties is not known in either category.

In the final days of the war, a Wehrmacht officer tore up the SS execution order for 160 prominent prisoners in the camp of Dachau, including Kállay and his friend, former French Prime Minister Léon Blum. He drove all of them to the nearest U.S. Army installation. Eventually U.S. authorities helped to set up Kállay in New York where he expressed to this writer, among others, his deep sorrow that his frequent wartime reminders to the Labor Service staff to respect "Hungary's traditional Christian values" had fallen on deaf ears.

In the post-war Republic of Hungary, controlled by Moscow, courts tended to hand down light punishments to those who tortured and executed Labor Service men.

The precise numbers may never be determined but it appears plausible that far more than 100,000 Jews, including Paul Ornstein and his father Lajos, were conscripted in the Labor Service and far more than 40,000 of them lost their lives there. Nevertheless, veterans of the Service were not prepared for a final tragedy: after the war's end, few of the men who returned home found their families still alive.

ACKNOWLEDGMENTS

My first and most heartfelt thanks go to Helen Epstein. Over the many years of our friendship, whenever I would reminisce about my childhood in a small town in Hungary or talk about my experiences in a Forced Labor Battalion in the Ukraine, Helen always paid close attention and wanted to hear more. In 2005, she began to record our conversations but it was not until 2015 that we decided that she would help me complete the psychoanalytic autobiography I wrote for a German publication (*Psychoanalyse in Selbstdarstellungen,* edited by Ludger M. Hermanns, Brandes & Apfel, 2007). Using additional source material (Jean Peck's *At the Fire's Center* and two published interviews with Jim Fish and Richard Geist), Helen gently but with persistence prodded my failing memory to remember details that I had long forgotten. I believe that this memoir would never have been written without her.

I also want to thank my wife for locating the pictures which tell the story in ways that words cannot express. Many thanks to Charles and Lizou Fenyvesi for providing an excellent historical context. I would also like to thank our many readers, Joseph Berger, Dr. Ira Brenner, Dr. Nancy Chodorow, Dr. Yehezkel Cohen, Dr. James Fisch, Dr. Eva Fogelman, Lester Lenoff, Dr. Judit Mészáros, Dr. Arnold Richards, Dr. Sophia Richman, Dr. Rachel Rosenblum, Dr. Michael Rosenbluth, Dr. Susannah Sherry and our three children: Drs. Sharone, Miriam and Rafael Ornstein.

GLOSSARY ~ Paul's glossary of non-English terms

aliyah is a Hebrew word that means "going up." It was used in two ways: to describe the honor of going up to read from the Torah during a religious service; and also to "go up" or emigrate to Palestine.

bar mitzvah: the ceremony for 13-year-old Jewish boys who are entering adult life (adult responsibilities).

bricha is a Hebrew word which literally means flight in the sense of escape. At that time, we used it to describe the process of getting to Palestine.

cheder: when I use the word *cheder*, I mean the place where I began my learning about Jewish and Hebrew subjects. It was one room not too far from my house, and there were about 10 to 12 boys — only boys, my age — who studied there.

daven: to daven means to pray in Yiddish.

erev is a Hebrew word meaning evening. All Jewish holidays (including *Shabbat*) begin on the evening before, i.e. *erev Shabbat.*

Festschrift: a term for a collection of scholarly papers in honor of a distinguished scholar.

hachsharah is a Hebrew term that means preparation. It refers to a process of preparing oneself to work in Palestine.

Hanukah: the Festival of Lights celebrating the ancient Jewish victory over the Greeks who wanted the Jews to worship their Gods.

kashrut refers to Biblical and Talmudic dietary prescriptions for orthodox Jews. It obliges Jews to separately eat dairy and meat, and consume only kosher products.

katyushas are Russian rockets that were fired at us during the Second World War.

mezuzah refers to a piece of Jewish scripture that is contained in a special box at the entry to a Jewish home, according to Jewish law.

midrash: a *midrash* is an explanation of a portion of the Bible by a Talmudic scholar.

shlemiel is the Yiddish word for nincompoop.

Shabbat is the Hebrew word for Sabbath.

shul is a Yiddish word that, in Hajdúnánás, means a small, plain building where Jews attended prayer services. In my town it was plain and small.

simulant is a pretender, usually someone who pretends to have an illness.

tallis is the Yiddish word for prayer shawl worn by orthodox Jews whenever they pray.

tzitzit is an undergarment with fringes that I wore under my shirt until I started Gymnasium. The religious Jews of Hajdúnánás let the fringes show from under their shirts as a mark of religiosity.

yeshiva, in Hajdúnánás, was the all-male Jewish alternative to Gymnasium, the school to which religious boys went after cheder in which they learned Talmud and other Jewish texts.

Yom Kippur: Day of Atonement.

PUBLICATIONS

1. **Ornstein PH**: An Experiment in Teaching Psychotherapy to Junior Medical Students *J. Med Educ.,* 36:2, 1961.

2. **Ornstein PH**, Whitman RM: Drug Therapy. In: Spiegel, EA (ed): Progress in Neurology and Psychiatry. New York: Grune & Stratton. Chap. 34, 631-658, 1963.

3. Whitman RM, **Ornstein PH**, Kramer M: Drug Therapy. In: Spiegel, EA (ed): Progress in Neurology and Psychiatry. New York: Grune & Stratton. Chap. 32, 606-630, 1964.

4. **Ornstein PH**: Evaluation of Newer Antidepressant Drugs. G.P. 30:91, 1964.

5. Whitman RM, **Ornstein PH**, Baldridge BJ: An Experimental Approach to the Psychoanalytic Theory of Dreams and Conflicts. *Compr. Psychiat.,* 5:349-363, 1964.

6. **Ornstein PH**, Whitman RM: On the Metapharmacology of Psychotropic Drugs. *Compr. Psychiat.,* 6:166-175, 1965.

7. Kramer M, **Ornstein PH**, Whitman RM: Drug Therapy. In: Spiegel, EA (ed): Progress in Neurology and Psychiatry, New York: Grune & Stratton. 33:723-753, 1965.

8. Kramer M, Whitman RM, Baldridge BJ, **Ornstein PH**: The Pharmacology of Dreaming, A Review. In: Enzymes in Mental Health, Martin GJ and Kisch B (Eds) Philadelphia, JB Lippincott. Chap. 8, 102-116, 1966.

9. **Ornstein PH**: Dreams and Conflicts. *Ohio State Med J,* 62:1271 -1280, 1966.

10. Whitman RM, Kramer M, **Ornstein PH**, Baldridge BJ: The Physiology, Psychology and Utilization of Dreams. *Amer J. Psychiat,* 124:287-302, 1967.

A. Whitman RM, Kramer M, Ornstein PH, Baldridge BJ:

The Physiology, Psychology and Utilization of Dreams. *Dig Neuro Psychiat,* 35:388, 1967.

11. Kramer M, **Ornstein PH**, Whitman RM, Baldridge BJ: The Contribution of Early Memories and Dreams to the Diagnostic Process. *Compr Psychiat,* 8: 344-374, 1967.

12. **Ornstein PH**, Kalthoff RJ: Toward a Conceptual Scheme for Teaching Clinical Psychiatric Evaluation. *Compr Psychiat,* 8:404-426, 1967.

13 **Ornstein PH**: Selected Problems in Learning How to Analyze. *Int. J. Psycho-Anal.,* 48:448-461, 1967.

14. Whitman RM, Kramer M, **Ornstein PH**, Baldridge BJ: The Influence of Drugs on Dreams. In: Herxheimer A (Ed.) Drugs and Sensory Functions. London, J&A Churchill. 299-329, 1968.

15. Baldridge BJ, Kramer M, Whitman RM, **Ornstein PH**: Smoking and Dreams. *Psychophys,* 4:372, 1968.

16. Kramer M, Whitman R, Baldridge B, **Ornstein PH**: Drugs and Dreams III: The Effects of Imipramine on the Dreams of the Depressed. *Amer J. Psychiat,* 124:1358-1392, 1968.

A. Kramer M, Whitman RM, Baldridge BJ, **Ornstein** PH: Imipramine: The Effects on the Dreams of the Depressed. *Psychophys,* 4:373, 1968.

B. Kramer M, Whitman RM, Baldridge BJ, **Ornstein PH**: Drugs and Dreams III: The Effects on the Dreams of the Depressed. *Psychiat Dig,* 29:43, 1968.

17. Fox RP, Kramer M, Whitman RM, **Ornstein PH**: The Experimenter Variable in Dream Research. *Dis Nerv Sys,* 29:698-701, 1968.

A. Fox RP, Kramer M, Whitman RM, **Ornstein PH**: The Experimenter Variable in Dream Research. *Psychophys,* 4:373, 1968.

18. Baldridge BJ, Kramer M, Whitman RM, **Ornstein PH**: University of Cincinnati Dream Scales. *Psychophys.,* 5:223, 1968.

19. Baldridge BJ, Kramer M, Whitman RM, **Ornstein PH**: The Effects of Induced Eye Movements on Dreaming. *Psychophys.,* 5:230, 1968.

20. **Ornstein PH**: What is and What is Not Psychotherapy? *Dis. Nerv. Sys.,* 29:118-123, 1968.

21. Baldridge BJ, Kramer M, Whitman RM, **Ornstein PH**: Self Associations of Schizophrenics. *Dis. Nerv. Sys.,* (Special Supplement), 29:124-128, 1968.

22. **Ornstein PH**: Sorcerer's Apprentice: The Initial Phase of Training in Psychiatry. In: Festschrift in Honor of Maurice Levine, M.D. *Compr. Psychiat.,* 9:293-315, 1968.

23. Kramer M, Whitman RM, Baldridge BJ, **Ornstein PH**: Drugs and Dreams HI. The Effects of Imipramine on the Dreams of the Depressed. *Amer J. Psychiat,* 124:1385-1392, 1968.

24. **Ornstein PH**: Trends in Psychoanalysis. *Ohio State Med J,* 64:1, 53-57, 1968.

25. Baldridge BJ, Whitman RM, Kramer M, **Ornstein PH**: Dual Chart Drive for Grass Polygraph. *Psychophys,* 5:440-443, 1969.

26. Kramer M, Baldridge BJ, Whitman RM, **Ornstein PH**, Smith PC: An Exploration of the Manifest Dream in Schizophrenic and Depressed Patients. *Dis. Nerv. Sys.,* 30:2, 126-130, 1969.

A. Kramer M, Baldridge BJ, Whitman RM, **Ornstein PH**, Smith PC: An Exploration of the Manifest Dream in Schizophrenic and Depressed Patients. *Psychophys,* 5:221, 1968.

B. Kramer M, Baldridge BJ, Whitman RM, **Ornstein PH**, Smith PC: An Exploration of the Manifest Dream in Schizophrenic and Depressed Patients. *Dig Neurol Psychiat,* 80, 1969.

27. **Ornstein PH**, Whitman RM, Kramer M, Baldridge BJ: Drugs and Dreams IV. Tranquilizers and Their Effects Upon Dreams and Dreaming in Schizophrenic Patients. *Exp Med Surg,* 27:145-156, 1969.

28. Whitman RM, Kramer M, **Ornstein PH**, Baldridge BJ: Drugs and Dream Content. *Exp. Med. Surg.,* 27:210-233, 1969.

29. Whitman RM, Kramer M, **Ornstein PH**, Baldridge BJ: Heart Rate Variability During Dreams and its Relationship to the Swallowing Reflex. *Psychophys.,* 5:484-584, 1969.

30. Kramer M, Whitman RM, Baldridge BJ, **Ornstein PH**: Dream Content in Schizophrenic Patients. *Psychophys.,* 6:249, 1969.

31. **Ornstein PH**: Discussion of Richard Jones' Ego Synthesis and Dreams: In: Dream Psychology and the New Biology of Dreaming. Kramer M (Ed.) with Whitman RM, Baldridge BJ. Springfield Illinois. Charles C Thomas, 1969.

32. Whitman RM, Kramer M, **Ornstein PH**, Baldridge BJ: The Varying Uses of the Dream in Clinical Psychiatry. In: The Psychodynamic Implications of the Physiological Studies on Dreams. Madow L, Snow LH (Eds.) Springfield Illinois. Charles C. Thomas, 1970.

33. **Ornstein PH**: In Memoriam Michael Balint 1896-1970. *Amer. J. Psychiat.,* 127:133, 1971.

34. **Ornstein PH**, Ornstein A: Focal Psychotherapy: Its Potential Impact on Psychotherapeutic Practice in Medicine. *Psychiatry in Medicine,* 3:311-325, 1972.

35. **Ornstein PH**, Goldberg A: Psychoanalysis and Medicine: I. Contributions to Psychiatry, Psychosomatic Medicine, and Medical Psychology. *Dis. Nerv. Sys.,* 34:143-147, 1973.

36. **Ornstein PH**, Goldberg A: Psychoanalysis and Medicine: II. Contributions to the Psychology of Medical Practice. *Dis. Nerv. Sys.,* 34:278-283, 1973.

37. **Ornstein PH**: A Discussion of the Paper by Otto F. Kernberg on "Further Contributions to the Psychoanalytic Treatment of Narcissistic Personalities". *Int. J. Psycho-Anal.* 55:241-247, 1974.

38. **Ornstein PH**: On Narcissism: Beyond the Introduction. Highlights of Heinz Kohut's Contributions to the Psychoanalytic

Treatment of Narcissistic Personality Disorders. *Annual of Psychoanalysis,* 2:127-149, 1974.

39. Ornstein A, **Ornstein PH**: On the Interpretive Process in Psychoanalysis. *Int. J. Psychoanal. Psychother.,* Langs R (Ed.) 4:219-271, Jason Aronson, New York, 1975.

40. **Ornstein PH**: Vitality and Relevance of Psychoanalytic Psychotherapy. *Compr. Psychiat.,* 16:6, 503-516, 1975.

41. **Ornstein PH**, Ornstein A, Lindy JD: On the Process of Becoming a Psychotherapist: An Outline of a Core-Curriculum for the Teaching and Learning of Psychoanalytic Psychotherapy. *Compr. Psychiat.,* 17:1, 177-190, 1976.

42. **Ornstein PH**: The Family Physician as a "Therapeutic Instrument". *The Journal of Family Practice,* 4:659-661, 1977.

43. **Ornstein PH**, Ornstein A: On the Continuing Evolution of Psychoanalytic Psychotherapy: Reflections and Predictions. *The Annual of Psychoanalysis,* Chicago Institute for Psychoanalysis, 5:329-370, International Universities Press, New York, 1977.

44. Ornstein A, **Ornstein PH**: Clinical Interpretations in Psychoanalysis. *International Encyclopedia of Neurology, Psychiatry and Psychology.* Wolman B (Ed.) 176-181, 1977.

45. **Ornstein PH**: The Resolution of a Mirror Transference: Clinical Emphasis Upon the Termination Phase. In: The Psychology of the Self: A Case Book. Goldberg A. (Ed.) International Universities Press, New York, 1978.

46. **Ornstein PH**: The Evolution of Heinz Kohut's Psychoanalytic Psychology of the Self. Introduction to Vols. I and II of The Search for the Self. Selected Writings of Heinz Kohut: 1950-1978. New York: International Universities Press. 1-106, 1978.

47. **Ornstein PH**: Remarks on the Central Position of Empathy in Psychoanalysis. *Bulletin: The Association for Psychoanalytic Medicine.* 18:95-109, 1979.

48. **Ornstein PH**: Self Psychology and the Concept of Health.

Publications

In: Advances in Self Psychology Goldberg A (ed.) International Universities Press, pp. 137-159, 1980.

Ornstein   PH: Der   Gesundheitsbegriff   der Selbstpsychologie. *Psychoanalyse.* 3:266-289, 1982.

49. **Ornstein PH**, Ornstein A: Formulating Interpretations in Clinical Psychoanalysis. *Int J. Psycho-Anal,* 61:203-211, 1980.

50. **Ornstein PH**: The Bipolar Self in the Psychoanalytic Treatment Process: Clinical-Theoretical Considerations. *J. Amer Psychoanal. Assoc.,* 29:353-375, 1981.

Ornstein PH: Il se bipolare nel processo di trattamento psicoanalitico: considerazione clinico-teoretiche. Gli Argonauti Psicoanalisi e Società, 17:105-122, 1983.

51. **Ornstein PH**, Ornstein A: Self Psychology and the Process or Regression. *Psychoanal. Inquiry,* 1:81-105, 1981.

52. **Ornstein PH**: On the Psychoanalytic Psychotherapy of Primary Self-Pathology. A Review and an Update. *Annual Review of Advances in Psychiatry,* 1982.

53. **Ornstein PH**: Discussion of: A Goldberg: "Self Psychology and Alternative Perspectives on Internalization", RD Stolorow: "Self Psychology — A Structural Psychology", RS Wallerstein: "Self Psychology and Classical Psychoanalytic Psychology: The Nature of Their Relationship — A Review and Overview". 339-384. In: Reflections on Self Psychology. Lichtenberg JD and Kaplan S (Eds.) Hillsdale, NJ, The Analytic Press, 1984.

54 **Ornstein PH**: Some Curative Factors and Processes in the Psychoanalytic Psychotherapies. 5:55-65, In: Cures by Psychotherapy: What. Effects Change? Meyers JM (Ed.) New York, Praeger, 198-4.

55. Ornstein A, **Ornstein PH**: Parenting as a Function of the Adult Sell": A Psychoanalytic Developmental Perspective. In: Parental Influences: In Health and Disease. Anthony J and Pollock G (Eds.) 181-231, 1985, Little Brown and Co.

56. **Ornstein PH**, Ornstein A: Clinical Understanding and

Explaining: The Empathic Vantage Point. In: Progress in Self Psychology. Goldberg A (Ed.) Vol. I 43-61, 1985. Guilford Press, New York.

57. **Ornstein PH**: The Thwarted Need to Grow: Clinical Theoretical Issues in the Self Object Transference. In: Transference in Psychotherapy, Clinical Management. Schwaber EA (Ed.). International Universities Press, 1986.

58. **Ornstein PH**: On Self State Dreams. In: The Interpretations of Dreams in Clinical Work. Rothstein A (Ed.). International Universities Press, 1987.

59. **Ornstein PH**: Multiple Curative Factors and Processes in the Psychoanalytic Psychotherapies. In: How Does Treatment Help? On the Modes of Therapeutic Action in Psychoanalytic Psychotherapy. Rothstein A (Ed.) International Universities Press, 1988.

60. **Ornstein PH**: The Fate of the Nuclear Self in the Middle Years. In: The Middle Years: New Psychoanalytic Perspectives. Oldham JM and Liebert RS (Eds.) Yale University Press. 1989.

Ornstein PH: Das Schicksal des Kernselbst in den mittleren Lebensjahren. In: Das Selbst im Lebenszyklus, pp. 85-99. Herausgegeben von HP Hartmann, W. E. Milch, Kutter, P. und Paal, J. Suhrkamp Taschenbuch Wissenshaft, 1998.

61. **Ornstein PH**, Kay J: Development of Psychoanalytic Self Psychology: A Historical Conceptual Overview. Chapter 16 In: Review of Psychiatry. Tasman A, Goldfinger SM, Kaufman CA (Eds.) Vol 9:303-322, 1990.

Ornstein PH: Die Entwicklung der Selbstpsychologie: Ein Historischer Ueberblick, pp. 27-42 In: Selbstpsychologie — Weiterentwicklungen nach Heinz Kohut. E.S. Wolf, A. Ornstein, P.H. Ornstein, J.D. Lichtenberg, P. Kutter. Verlag Internationale Psychoanalyse, 1989.

Ornstein PH, Kay J: Lo Sviluppo Delia Psicologia Psicoanalitica Del Se: Una Panoramica Sorico-Concettuale. Edizioni Universitarie Romane, 1993.

Publications

62. Ornstein A, **Ornstein PH**: The Process of Psychoanalytic Psychotherapy: A Self Psychological Perspective. Chapter 17 In: Review of Psychiatry. Tasman A, Goldfinger SM, Kaufman, CA (Eds.) Vol. 9:323-340, 1990.

63. **Ornstein PH**: A Case Discussion: The Self Psychology Perspective. Chapter 6 In: New Perspectives on Narcissism. Plakun EM (Ed.) American Psychiatric Press, Inc. 205-252, 199.

64. **Ornstein PH**: How to Enter a Psychoanalytic Process Conducted by Another Analyst. *Psychoanal. Inquiry,* 10:478-497, 1990.

65. **Ornstein PH**: The Unfolding and Completion of Heinz Kohut's Paradigm of Psychoanalysis. Introduction to Vols. III and IV In: The Search for the Self. Selected Writings of Heinz Kohut: 1978-1981. Madison, CT, International Universities Press, pp. 1-78, 1990.

66. **Ornstein PH**: From Narcissism to Ego Psychology to Self Psychology. In: Freud's On Narcissism: An Introduction. Sandler J, Person ES, Fonagy P (Eds.) International Psychoanalytic Association. Yale University Press. 175-194, 1991.

67. **Ornstein PH**: Why Self Psychology Is Not an Object Relations Theory: Clinical and Theoretical Considerations. Chapter 2 In: The Evolution of Self Psychology — Progress in Self Psychology. Goldberg A (Ed.) The Analytic Press. Hillsdale, NJ. 7:17-29, 1991.

68. **Ornstein PH**: A Self Psychological Perspective on Conflict and Compromise. Chapter 10 In: Conflict and Compromise: Therapeutic Implications. Monograph Seven. Workshop Series of The American Psychoanalytic Association. Dowling S (Ed.) The International Universities Press. Madison CT, pp. 133-171, 1991.

69. **Ornstein PH**: How to Read The Basic Fault? An Introduction to Michael Balint's Seminal Ideas on the Psychoanalytic Treatment Process, pp. vii-xxv In: Michael Balint, The Basic Fault. Northwestern University Press, Evanston, Ill.,

1992.

70. **Ornstein PH** and Ornstein, A: Assertiveness, Anger, Rage, and Destructive Aggression: A Perspective from the Treatment Process. In: "Rage, Power, and Aggression, (eds.) Glick, R. A. and Roose, S. P., Yale University Press, New Haven, CT, 1993.

Ornstein, PH and Ornstein, A.: Selbstbehauptung, Aerger, Wut und zerstorerishe Aggression. Psyche: 51:289-310, April, 1997.

71. Ornstein A and **Ornstein PH**: Empatia e Dialogo Terapeutico. Edizione Universitarie Romane, 1993.

72. **Ornstein PH**: Chronic Rage From Underground: Reflections on its Structure and Treatment. In: The Widening Scope of Self Psychology: Progress in Self Psychology, Vol. 9, (ed) A. Goldberg, Hillsdale, NJ: The Analytic Press, pp. 143-157, 1993.

Ornstein PH: La Rabbia Cronica Dal "Sotto-Suolo": Riflessioni Sulla Struttura E Sul Trattamento. *Attualità in Psicologia.* 8:14-24, 1993.

73. **Ornstein PH**: Is Self Psychology on a Promising Trajectory? Some Personal Reflections. In: The Widening Scope of Self Psychology: Progress in Self Psychology, Goldberg, Hillsdale, NJ: The Analytic Press, Vol. 9 pp. 1-11, 1993.

74. **Ornstein PH**: Sexuality and Aggression in Pathogenesis and in the Clinical Situation. In: The Widening Scope of Self Psychology: Progress in Self Psychology, Vol. 9, (ed) A. Goldberg, Hillsdale, NJ: The Analytic Press, pp. 109-125, 1993.

Ornstein PH: Zur Bedeutung von Sexualitaet und Aggression fuer die Pathogenese psychischer Erkrankungen, pp. 77-97. In: Sexualitaet und Aggression aus der Sicht der Selbstpsycholgie. Herausgegeben von Ch. Schoettler und P. Kutter. Suhrkamp Taschenbuch, 1992.

75. **Ornstein PH**: Did Freud Understand Dora? In "Freud's Case Studies: Self-Psychological Perspectives." (ed) Barry

Magid. The Analytic Press, Hillsdale, NJ, 1993.

76. **Ornstein PH**: The Clinical Impact of the Psychotherapist's View of Human Nature. Journal of Psychotherapy Practice and Research, 2:193-204, 1993.

77. **Ornstein PH**, Ornstein, A.: On The Conceptualization of Clinical Facts in Psychoanalysis. *Int. J. Psycho-Anal.* 75:977-994, 1994.

78. **Ornstein PH**: Psychoanalysis in Search of a Pedagogy. Newsletter, The American Psychoanalytic Association.

79. **Ornstein PH**, Ornstein, A: Some Distinguishing Features of Heinz Kohut's Self Psychology. *Psychoanalytic Dialogues,* 5:385-391, 1995.

80. Ornstein A, **Ornstein PH**: Marginal Comments on the Evolution of Self Psychology. *Psychoanalytic Dialogues,* 5:421-425, 1995.

81. **Ornstein PH**: Self Psychology Is Not What You Think It Is. *Journal of Clinical Psychoanalysis,* 4:491-506, 1995.

82. **Ornstein PH**: Introduction to "Classic Articles:" Heinz Kohut's "Introspection Empathy and Psychoanalysis: An Examination of the Relationship Between Mode of Observation and Theory." *Journal of Psychotherapy Practice and Research* 4:159-162, 1995.

83. **Ornstein PH**: Critical Reflections on a Comparative Analysis of Self Psychology and Intersubjectivity Theory. In: *The Impact of New Ideas — Progress in Self Psychology* 11:47-77, 1995.

84. **Ornstein PH**, Ornstein, A.: I. Some General Principles of Psychoanalytic Psychotherapy: A Self-Psychological Perspective. In *Understanding Therapeutic Action: Psychodynamic Concepts of Cure.* (Ed) Lifson, L. E., Hillsdale, NJ: The Analytic Press, Inc. pp. 87-101, 1996.

85. Ornstein, A. **Ornstein PH**: II. Speaking in the Interpretive Mode and Feeling Understood: Crucial Aspects of the Therapeutic Action in Psychotherapy. In *Understanding*

Therapeutic Action: Psychodynamic Concepts of Cure. (Ed.) Lifson, L.E., Hillsdale, NJ: The Analytic Press, Inc. pp. 103-125, 1996.

86. **Ornstein PH**: Heinz Kohut's Legacy. *Partisan Review,* Vol. LXIII:614-626, 1996.

87. **Ornstein PH**: Heinz Kohut's Vision of the Essence of Humanness. In *Psychoanalytic Versions of the Human Condition and Clinical Practice.* (Eds.) Marcus, P. Rosenberg, A. New York: New York University Press, 1998.

88. **Ornstein PH**: Omnipotence in Health and Illness: A Perspective from Everyday Life and the Psychoanalytic Treatment Process. In: *Omnipotent Fantasies and the Vulnerable Self,* (eds) Ellman, C. and Reppen, J. New Jersey: Jason Aronson, Inc. 1997.

89. **Ornstein PH**: Psychoanalysis of Patients With Primary Self-Disorder: A Self Psychological Perspective. In: The American Psychiatric Press, 1997.

90. **Ornstein PH** and Jerald Kay: "Enduring Difficulties in Medical Education and Training: Is There a Cure?" *The Annual of Psychoanalysis,* (ed.) J. A. Winer. Hillsdale, NJ, The Analytic Press, Vol. XXV: pp. 155-172, 1997.

91. **Ornstein PH**: Foreword to Juan-David Nasio's *"Hysteria or The Splendid Child of Psychoanalysis"* pp. XVII-XXII, Northvale, NJ: Jason Aronson, 1997.

92. **Ornstein PH**: On the Function of Theory in the Interpretive Process in Psychoanalysis.

93. **Ornstein PH**: Schicksale des Deutungsprozesses in der psychoanalytischen Beziehung In: *Die Deutung im Therapeutischen Prozess,* (Hg) W.E. Milch, H-P. Hartmann. Bibliothek der Psychoanalyse-Giessen: Psychosozial-Verlag, 1999.

94. **Ornstein PH**, Ornstein, A.: Der Einfluss der Selbstpsychologie auf die Durchfuerung und den Prozess der psychoanalytischen Psychotherapie. In: Selbstpsycholgie:

Europaeishe Zeitschrift fuer Psychoanalytische Therapie in Forschung. 1. JG. pp. 161-178. Heft 2, 2000.

95. Ornstein, A, **Ornstein, PH**: Alle "guten" psychoanalytischen Psychotherapien sind supportive — und was zeichnet "gute" Psychotherapien aus? Psychotherapie in Psychiatrie, Psychotherapeutischer Medizin und Klinischer Psychologie, pp. 186-196, JG. 5, Band 5, Heft 2, 2000.

96. **Ornstein PH**, Ornstein, A.: The Function of Theory in Psychoanalysis: A Self Psychological Perspective. P.Q., Vol. LXXII, pp. 157-182, 2003.

97. **Ornstein PH**: The Elusive Concept of the Psychoanalytic Process. JAPA, 52:15-41, 2004.

98. **Ornstein PH** and Anna Ornstein: The Function of Theory in Psychoanalysis: A Self Psychological Perspective. Psychoanal. Q. 72:157-182, 2003.

99. Ornstein, A. and **Ornstein, PH**: Conflict in Contemporary Clinical Work: A Self Psychological Perspective. Psychoanal. Q. 74: 219-251, 2005.

100. **Ornstein PH**: When "Dora" Came to See Me for a Second Analysis. *Psychoanal. Inquiry.* 25:94-114, 2005.

101. **Ornstein, PH** & Ornstein, A. (2008): The Structure and Function of Unconscious Fantasy in the Psychoanalytic Treatment Process, *Psychoanal. Inquiry,* 28:206-230.

102. **Ornstein, PH** (2008): Multiple Narratives of the Origin of Kohut's Self Psychol. *Am. Imago* 65:567-584.

103. **Ornstein, PH** (2009): A comparative assessment of an analysis of envy. Commentary on paper by Julie Gerhardt, *Psychoanal. Dialogue* 19:309-317.

104. **Ornstein, PH** (2009): My Late Night Hypnogogic Fantasy: Conversations with Heinz Kohut, *Int. J. Psychoanal. Self Psychology* 4:101-110.

105. **Ornstein, PH** (2011): The Centrality of Empathy in Psychoanalysis *Psychoanal. Inquiry* 31:437-447.

Publications

106. **Ornstein, PH** (2012): The Novelist's Craft: Reflections on the Brothers Karamazov, *Am. Imago* 69:295-317.

107. **Ornstein, PH** (2015): On Choosing a Guiding Theory for Treatment in a Pluralistic Psychoanalytic World: My Personal Journey. *Int. J. Psychoanal. Self Psych.* 10:107-117.

108. **Ornstein, PH** (2015): Revisiting the negative therapeutic reaction: an example of comparative psychoanalysis. *Int. J. Psychoanal. Self Psychol.* 10:118-127.

BOOKS

1. Balint M, **Ornstein PH**, Balint E.: Focal Psychotherapy: An Example of Applied Psychoanalysis. London: Tavistock Publications and Philadelphia, Lippincott, 1972.

2. Ornstein A. and **Ornstein, PH**: Empathie und Therapeutischer Dialog: Beitraege zur klinischen Praxis der psychoanalytischen Selbstpsychologie. Psychosozial-Verlag, Giessen Germany, 2001.

3. **Ornstein, PH**: The search for the self: selected writings of Heinz Kohut. Vol 1-2, 1950-1978. Vol 3-4, 1978-1981, International Universities Press, 1990-1.

Paul Ornstein was born in Hajdúnánás, Hungary in 1924 and educated at the Franz Josef Rabbinical Seminary in Budapest, where he discovered psychoanalysis. After surviving the Shoah in Hungary, he received his degree in medicine from the University of Heidelberg, then emigrated to the United States and became a leading figure in psychoanalytic self-psychology. Dr. Ornstein is a graduate of the Chicago Institute for Psychoanalysis, an Emeritus Professor of Psychiatry and Psychoanalysis at the University of Cincinnati Medical School, and a Supervising Analyst at the Boston Psychoanalytic Institute. He co-authored *Focal Psychotherapy: An Example of Applied Psychoanalysis* with Michael and Enid Balint and edited *The Search for the Self: selected writings of Heinz Kohut*.

Helen Epstein (www.helenepstein.com) was born in Prague in 1947 and was educated in New York City and Jerusalem. A veteran journalist, she is the author of the books *Children of the Holocaust*, *Where She Came From*, *Joe Papp* and *Music Talks*, editor of *Archivist on a Bicycle*, and translator from the Czech of Heda Kovály's *Under A Cruel Star* and Vlasta Schönová's *Acting in Terezín*.

Charles Fenyvesi was born in Debrecen, Hungary in 1937. He is a former *Washington Post* staff writer and *U.S. News & World Report* columnist who has written six nonfiction books, including *When Angels Fooled the World* and *When the World Was Whole*.

Other titles from Plunkett Lake Press
available as eBooks

By **Inge Deutschkron**
Outcast: A Jewish Girl in Wartime Berlin

By **Helen Epstein**
Children of the Holocaust
Where She Came From: A Daughter's Search for Her
Mother's History

By **Charles Fenyvesi**
When The World Was Whole: Three Centuries of
Memories

By **Sebastian Haffner**
Defying Hitler: A Memoir
The Meaning of Hitler

By **Eva Hoffman**
Lost in Translation

By **Ernest Jones**
The Life and Work of Sigmund Freud

By **Heda Margolius Kovály**
Under A Cruel Star: A Life in Prague, 1941-1968

By **Susan Quinn**
A Mind of Her Own: The Life of Karen Horney

By **Susan Rubin Suleiman**
Budapest Diary: In Search of the Motherbook

By **Joseph Wechsberg**
The Vienna I Knew: Memories of a European Childhood

By **Chaim Weizmann**
Trial and Error: The Autobiography of Chaim Weizmann

By **Charlotte Wolff**
Hindsight: An Autobiography

By **Stefan Zweig**
Freud by Zweig
Mental Healers: Franz Anton Mesmer, Mary Baker Eddy, Sigmund Freud
The World of Yesterday

For more information, visit www.plunkettlakepress.com

Made in the USA
Middletown, DE
22 March 2016